Menopause

Menopause

Natural and medical solutions

Kaz Cooke
& Ruth Trickey

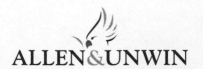

ALLEN&UNWIN

Thanks to Gemma Ridgeway-Faye for editing assistance on this series.

Allen & Unwin
83 Alexander Street
Crows Nest NSW 2065
Australia
Phone: (61 2) 8425 0100
Fax: (61 2) 9906 2218
Email: info@allenandunwin.com
Web: www.allenandunwin.com

National Library of Australia
Cataloguing-in-Publication entry:

Cooke, Kaz, 1962- .
    Menopause : natural and medical solutions.

    Includes index.
    ISBN 1 86508 763 7.

    1. Menopause. 2. Menopause - Treatment. 3. Menopause -
Alternative treatment. I. Trickey, Ruth, 1953- .
    II. Title.

618.17506

Cover and text design by Dianna Wells Design
Set in 12/14 pt MrsEavesRoman by Bookhouse, Sydney
Printed in Australia by McPherson's Printing Group

10 9 8 7 6 5 4 3 2

Contents

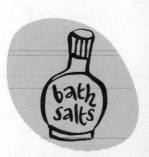

ABOUT THE AUTHORS

Ruth Trickey is a herbalist with a medical background. She specialises in the application of Chinese and European herbal treatments of women's health problems. She runs the Melbourne Holistic Health Group in Melbourne, and treats many patients in conjunction with their doctors and surgeons. Ruth is the author of *Women, Hormones and The Menstrual Cycle*, and a frequent lecturer and guest speaker in Australia, New Zealand, Europe and North America.

Kaz Cooke is a cartoonist and author. She is the author of *Real Gorgeous: The Truth about Body and Beauty*; *Up the Duff: The Real Guide to Pregnancy*; *Living with Crazy Buttocks*; a children's book called *The Terrible Underpants* and the satirical *Little Book of . . .* series, encompassing *Stress*, *Dumb Feng Shui*, *Household Madness*, *Beauty*, and *Diet and Exercise*.
www.kazcooke.com

Most of the information in this small book is edited and updated from the text of *Women's Trouble*, by the same authors, also published by Allen & Unwin. Also in this series of small books on women's health: *Endometriosis* and *Problem Periods*.

All advice given in this book is general and not intended to be used instead of professional medical advice. Any of the advice herein should be undertaken only after consultation with your doctor and natural therapies practitioner. Each person in your advice team must be aware of all drugs, herbs and other treatments you are undergoing. It is not safe to self-diagnose, or self-prescribe with either herbs or drugs. Individual and tailored treatments can only be obtained from your own practitioners.

Intro

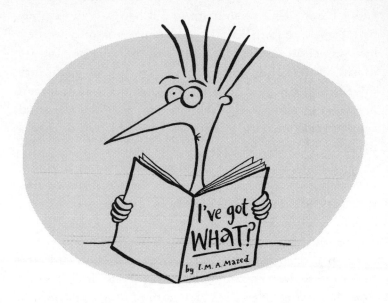

The typical stereotype of a 'menopausal woman' is a neurotic, grumpy old bag plagued by insomnia, struggling through her day being constantly overwhelmed and humiliated by hot flushes that leave her feeling faint, sweating like a maniac and liable to whack somebody over the noggin with her handbag. Well on her way to needing those adult nappies they advertise so coyly, she couldn't be bothered with sex, young people, or new-fangled ways of cooking peas. In some people's minds, menopause is even linked with dementia.

The real 'typical' menopausal woman may have some temporary problems with menopausal complaints like hot flushes, but they don't stop her from getting on with her life. Being in your late forties or 50-something isn't old (no it bloody isn't so shut up or I'll have at you with my handbag), but for all sorts of complex reasons, women have somehow confused ageing and menopause. Images of old women often show them as fearful, or gossiping, or senile. Many people lump together the years between menopause and death with the tag 'post-menopausal woman'; they imagine a batty 98-year-old, rather than a dynamic 50-, 60- or even 70-year-old.

And of course there's the implication that if you've got wrinkles, they're not beautiful character lines tracing a history of life and accumulated experience, but an appalling misbehaviour in the Trying To Look Like A Supermodel stakes. Getting 'old' is seen as a bad career move in a society which worships youth. We don't all long to be 50 so we can look like Susan Sarandon, despite those ludicrous captions underneath photographs of Miss Sarandon suggesting she's a flagbearer for the woman in her 50s. I suspect that Miss Sarandon looks about 28 not because of a simple spiritual serenity. I think make-up, lighting, computer enhancements, and call me crazy, possibly even a little surgery may have taken place (I'm only guessing). The more common message absorbed is why don't you look like this when you're over 50? All this can build up a fear of ageing.

Making menopause a time of positive change rather than a major freakout is a matter of planning. Preparing for mid-life with a good diet, lifestyle, exercise program

and especially attitude, will determine how you experience menopause—and what comes after. Some people feel
somewhat relieved that they no longer have to be seen as
sexual beings, or even liberated from their childbearing
or relentless menstruating years and seeing a new lease
of sexual life. Many women feel 'the change' empowers
them and lets them please themselves more. Others are
terrified of any 'changes' and want to take hormone
replacement therapy until they're 90.

WHAT IS MENOPAUSE, EXACTLY?

Menopause literally means stopping menstruation. The
word is made up of the trusty, rusty old Greek: *meno*
(monthly) and *pausis* (to stop). You won't know
menopause has happened until a whole year has passed
since the date of your last period—the actual date can only
be decided retrospectively, by counting backwards.
Medically recognised menopause actually happens on one
distinct date (forget Tupperware, now you can have a
menopause party).

The medical term for what we usually mean by 'menopausal' or 'going through the menopause' is 'climacteric',
or 'peri-menopausal'. The peri-menopause, like puberty
and the years when the menstrual cycle starts to become
established, is characterised by irregular periods, hormonal fluctuation, and sometimes, an emotional
roller-coaster. We're just going to call it 'menopausal',
because most people do.

WHEN TO EXPECT IT

Menopause between the ages of 45 and 55 is considered normal. Most women in Australia become menopausal between 48 and 53. Thinner women are much more likely to have an earlier menopause than women who are heavier. Being very overweight can delay the onset of menopause until well into the fifties.

Early menopause

Premature menopause is when you have your last period before you're 40. The ovaries, which release the hormones and eggs which drive the menstrual cycle, stop working before the usual time. Menopause may deliberately be brought on for medical reasons, or accidentally triggered by surgery, some drugs or illness. Nobody really knows why some women's ovaries suddenly take early retirement. Some people say it happened to them during a period of extreme stress. Another theory is that the body makes a mistake and produces antibodies to ovarian tissue, causing premature ovarian shut-down. Auto-immune diseases, and in rare cases, mumps can also bring on the menopause. Early menopause is often overlooked by doctors looking for a diagnosis in younger women.

Medically-induced menopause

Relatively new drugs can bring on a 'temporary menopause' in treating some cases of endometriosis and uterine fibroids. These drugs are called gonadotrophin releasing hormone agonists (GnRH agonists). The most common brand is Zoladex.

The menopausal state is reversed when the drugs are stopped. While on the drugs, the changes are usually the same as any natural menopause: bone density loss, vaginal dryness, hot flushes and mood changes. Although the condition can be reversed, it can be much harder to regain the bone density once off the drugs. Menopause can also come on after radiation therapy for cancer, particularly of the pelvis. Sometimes this is not deliberate, but the changes are often permanent. The ovarian tissue degenerates and fails to work in the usual way, and menopause is the result. The herb *Angelica sinensis* (Dang Gui) may help to protect the ovaries from the effects of irradiation. It must be properly prescribed by a herbalist.

Some drugs used in the treatment of cancer are of necessity pretty strong stuff. They include cyclophosphamide, chlorambucil, mechlorethamine and vincristine. These drugs can potentially cause menopausal symptoms and their use may be associated with permanent infertility and menopause. Tamoxifen, used as an antioestrogen in the treatment of breast cancer, can also cause menopause-like symptoms.

Surgically-induced menopause

Surgically-induced menopause is rarer now that drugs achieve the same result. In the past, it was more common to have a hysterectomy in which the ovaries and uterus were both surgically removed. (If you let them, surgeons will refer to this as a bilateral salpingo-oophorectomy.) This operation, or the surgical removal of the ovaries only, will immediately create a menopausal state. This type of surgery may be performed for very severe endometriosis, oestrogen-dependent breast cancer, ovarian tumours or ovarian cancer.

According to conventional medical wisdom, a hysterectomy which takes the uterus and leaves the ovaries shouldn't cause any interruption in ovarian activity—but up to one-third of women who have this surgery do have menopausal symptoms. If menopause isn't brought on immediately by a hysterectomy, it will arrive an average of five years earlier than in women who still have their uterus. One theory is that ovarian shut-down can happen earlier because of the alteration in ovarian blood supply after the surgery. Another controversial, unproven theory claims that tubal ligation ('having your tubes tied') may also be associated with premature menopause for much the same reasons.

NORMAL STAGE OR A DISEASE?

Some doctors believe menopause is a 'deficiency' disease, characterised by a lack of oestrogen, and comparable to other disorders caused by hormone deficiency such as diabetes, Cushing's disease and hypothyroidism. Hormone deficiency diseases, they claim, are states which can be reversed or held off by replacing a hormone. This mob says that medication should replace the deficient hormone and return the body to 'normal'. They are big fans of hormone replacement therapy (HRT) and believe that all post-menopausal women, having outlived the functional lives of their ovaries, are diseased and in need of continued medical attention until they die.

For these doctors, menopause is just like other

 6

hormonal disorders, such as diabetes, but has the peculiarity of affecting all women at about the same time in their lives. It's a bit much to say that every single one of us is biologically faulty and in need of treatment and medication. (Not to mention a Bex and a good lie down.)

Some doctors have introduced an air of vagueness and contradiction into this debate. In her book for the mid-life woman, *Menopause*, Dr Miriam Stoppard writes 'While I believe that the menopause is a normal stage in a woman's life, I also believe that it is a true deficiency state . . .' She also endorses hormone replacement therapy (we'll get to HRT later . . .).

Most natural therapists and many doctors view menopause as a normal transition, although people may need supportive treatment for any rogue symptoms. Rather than telling all mid-life women they are diseased, these practitioners encourage menopausal women to adopt positive lifestyle changes, good eating patterns and a positive attitude to the changes.

POSITIVE THINKING

Researchers in one study found that levels of hormones were not the relevant factor in what sort of menopause a woman had. The important elements were being physically well, exercising moderately, having a positive attitude to menopause and feeling happy. Exercising, even once a week, was associated with fewer menopausal 'side effects', and so were positive relationships and friendships. Changing your diet can reduce some menopausal symptoms.

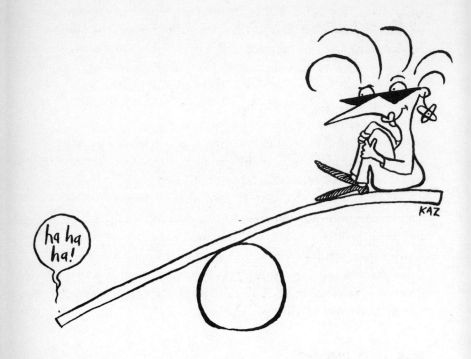

Balancing the hormones

 8

The Changes

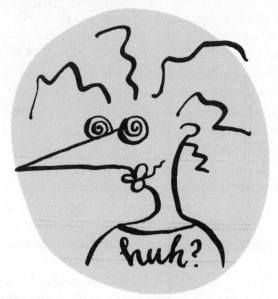

THE HORMONES

All the time, inside us, we produce varying levels of the sex hormones which set up a regular menstrual cycle. You seething sexual being, you. There's a lot going on, with various departments at work. At any time during the menstrual cycle, wee eggs are hanging around—some ready to be released down the tubes, some getting ready, some just starting and some disintegrating. Technically speaking, the developing egg is called a follicle and the mature egg is called an ovum.

9

This goes on with rather tedious regularity for years and years, as long as you're ovulating. As menopause approaches, the follicles are less responsive to the hormonal stimulation, and the body makes fewer of the hormones. The ovaries have fewer eggs-in-waiting left, and eventually no more of them will go on to produce ova.

As you approach menopause you might also have an irregular cycle because there are fewer eggs being made and because the hormonal feedback loop slows down, so ovulation isn't triggered so regularly, or in the end, at all. Stress is also more likely to get in the way of a regular cycle around the time of the menopause.

Every month after the period, the ovaries start to secrete active oestrogen called oestradiol (pronounced east-rar-dye-al). Some of the oestradiol is converted into a weaker oestrogen called oestrone (east-rone), and then both oestradiol and oestrone go on a trip together in the bloodstream, travelling to exotic lands . . . sorry. They travel to oestrogen-sensitive cells to stimulate cell growth. The ovaries pump out the most oestrogen after ovulation, and cut back just before the period. Meanwhile, the body makes a second source of oestrone from androgen hormones. This process, using an enzyme, is referred to as 'peripheral conversion' or 'aromatisation'. Aromatisation happens in the hair follicles, the skin, the brain, bone and bone marrow, muscle and fatty tissue. About 25 per cent of the conversion goes on in the muscle and 10–15 per cent in the fat. After the menopause, we make almost all our oestrogen from aromatisation, as our ovaries 'retire'.

The 'oestrogen pool'

Sounds like a rather good name for a sexy nightclub, but it refers to the range of oestrogens available for use by the body. There are many factors that cause oestrogenic effects which can come from outside the body. These include the phyto-oestrogens produced in plants, which are good for you, and the much more dangerous 'environmental oestrogens', which are consumed as hormones added to foods or as containments of foods, such as pesticides. All of these different types of 'oestrogens' can have oestrogen-like activities in the body.

An oestrogenic effect is caused by any substance which has the ability to connect to an oestrogen receptor site. It has to be said, quite frankly, that oestrogen receptor sites are pretty stupid, and will often accept any substance which has a molecular similarity to the oestrogen produced in the body, even if it's a chemical pesticide.

The receptor sites can be monopolised by oestrogen-like substance from plants which don't have a very strong oestrogenic effect. The substances have, in a way, taken most of the oestrogen parking spaces. The stronger oestrogens, made in the body, can't get as many parks, so they can't go to work and do their stuff.

In this way the body can be exposed to a weaker combination of oestrogens. Before menopause, this can help protect against the disorders linked to having too much oestrogen.

After menopause, when you're not making so much oestrogen in your own body because your ovaries have 'retired', plant oestrogens or oestrogenic herbs can help

11

fill all the empty parking spaces and help boost your depleted 'oestrogen pool'.

HORMONE LEVELS

The hormonal changes usually come on slowly. About two to three years before ovulation stops, levels of oestrogen and progesterone decline gradually, sometimes in association with irregular periods. When hormone production changes gradually, fewer menopausal symptoms may be the result. (This may be one reason why 'naturally' menopausal women tend to have a much easier time of it than women who get the menopause in one big hit brought on by surgery or drugs, or an early end to ovary function.) Lots of hormonal variations, not just declining oestrogen, cause physical and biochemical changes. The most common ones include changes in the menstrual cycle, hot flushes and the dreaded PMS-type mood swings.

FSH and LH

Basically what happens is that the ovaries which run the menstrual show start to retire and this results in the changes in hormone balance. During the menstrual cycle, oestrogen usually holds down levels of follicle stimulating hormone (FSH). As oestrogen declines, the FSH level rises. (FSH levels in blood are sometimes used as a biochemical indicator of menopause.) Luteinising hormone (LH) also increases. Both LH and FSH are released in small bursts about every hour to an hour and a half. It has been shown that the 'bursts' of LH coincide with hot flushes.

Oestrogen

The dominant kind of oestrogen in post-menopausal women is oestrone. This is converted from androgens in the fatty tissues, because the ovaries have stopped making oestradiol. Oestrone is weaker than oestradiol but is still thought to contribute to the increased bone density and lack of menopausal symptoms experienced by 'heavier' women with a higher percentage of body fat or muscle bulk.

Testosterone

After menopause, the ovaries continue producing some testosterone as has always been the case. Testosterone is an androgen (male hormone) and is probably responsible for some of the facial hair and male-pattern baldness in some post-menopausal women. Oestrogen would normally balance it all out. To offset the effects of this continued testosterone, you need more sex hormone binding globulin (SHBG), a carrier protein. Vegetarian diets and diets with a high plant oestrogen content increase SHBG. (The plant oestrogen diet info is in the Self Care chapter.)

Lately however, doctors have been increasingly prescribing testosterone with HRT to improve libido in those women who experience low sex drive after menopause. These are new treatments and are discussed in the HRT section.

Progesterone

Progesterone, the other big star of girly hormones, is the building block for many of the other steroid hormones. So it plays an important role not only in periods and reproduction, but also in a number of other jobs in the body. It stimulates changes in organs with progesterone-sensitive tissue. In the uterus, progesterone stimulates the endometrium so that it can support a developing embryo. If the egg is not fertilised, the level of progesterone falls, the endometrial tissue disintegrates and is shed as a period.

Progesterone initiates glandular changes in breast tissue so that the breast is capable of giving milk. It also keeps the normal female levels of androgen (blokey) hormones in check. Progesterone production slows or stops after menopause, and androgen levels increase. This may account for hair falling out of the head but mysteriously turning up on the chin when some of us get older.

Progesterone has other actions that include improved fat metabolism, an increase in bone density, good moods, and a natural diuretic (fluid loss) effect. It also helps to prevent both cancerous and benign breast changes by counterbalancing the effects of oestrogen in the breast, and has the same protective and counterbalancing effect on the endometrium. Progesterone is also the building block of the hormones called corticosteroids which maintain stable blood sugar levels, reduce inflammation and help the body fight the effects of stress.

Progesterone production is all over the shop around the menopause because ovulation happens less often and less regularly. This may contribute to mood changes, especially before the period.

MENSTRUAL CYCLE CHANGES

Before menopause, the menstrual cycle is usually regular and the period flow is one you're used to. Many women notice changes in the period flow or its regularity. The period may come more often (which is very boring), but more often the cycle length increases because ovulation is winding down. This means you still get periods, but at longer and longer intervals. This stage may last for a few months or for a few years. During this phase, you might think it's all over (there's a list below of other problems that can cause menopause-like symptoms), but be warned: you can still get pregnant. The most important thing to remember for women who think they're approaching 'the change' and don't want to be a later-life parent or face a much higher statistical chance of miscarriage or a damaged child: KEEP USING CONTRACEPTION, even if you think you're period's erratic, or even stopped, until you get a medical diagnosis of true menopause. You wouldn't believe how many women in their late forties and early fifties have pregnancy scares. It just isn't worth it.

Other changes in your cycle can include heavier periods, hot flushes and night sweats. Blame your oestrogen levels. Some women stop having periods all of a sudden; others may have normal periods further apart; some have surprise 'flooding': heavy bleeding. This is sometimes referred to as the 'transitional phase' because

15

it represents the stage immediately before menopause. Finally, periods stop completely and you become officially menopausal.

WHAT YOU'LL BE MISSING

What exactly is a period anyway?

A period is the regular shedding of the endometrium—the lining of the uterus—once every month for most of us. It looks like blood, and we call it blood, but it's made up of other tissues and secretions as well as blood, from the inside of the uterus. Most textbooks and doctors talk about periods in relation to pregnancy: 'Ahem. If pregnancy does not occur, menstruation will commence', with the implication that pregnancy is the usual event and a period is the second prize. Some melodramatic male authors even used to refer to periods as 'the weeping womb'.

Many of us, though, don't think of a period as a missed opportunity to conceive, but rather as a relief because there's no pregnancy.

WRONG DIAGNOSIS

Something you might mistake for menopause is not enough oestrogen. You may start having erratic cycles, no periods or menopause-like symptoms, such as hot flushes if your oestrogen is too low. A relative oestrogen deficiency happens when:

- too much oestrogen is cleared by the body
- too little is recycled for use by the body

- and/or the fat cells aren't making enough oestrogen from the androgen hormones.

An actual oestrogen deficiency happens after menopause, when your ovaries stop making it.

Symptoms
Low bone density, poor fertility, low sex drive, irregular periods, and premature ageing or excessive dryness and brittleness of tissues including vagina, bones and skin.

Possible causes
- Body weight 15–20 per cent below the recommended range of the body mass index (BMI) can often stop periods and cause oestrogen levels to fall below normal. To see if your body weight is in the normal range for your height you can calculate your BMI by dividing your weight in kilograms by your height in centimetres squared.

  For example, if you weigh 52 kilos and your height is 1.7 metres, you divide the weight (52) by the square of your height (1.7 times 1.7 is 2.89). The answer to the calculation is 17.99. Rounded up to the nearest full number, your BMI is 18, and that puts you in the underweight category.

  Roughly speaking, on the BMI scale:
  - Less than 20 is considered to be underweight.
  - 20–25 is normal.
  - 26–30 is overweight.
  - Over 30 is considered to be obese.

  The BMI is only a guide, and if your body frame

is very slight or very large, give yourself a bit of latitude. If you are underweight the cycle can also become erratic, and fertility and bone density are also reduced.

- Too much fibre lowers oestrogen levels and may increase your chances of developing osteoporosis. Avoid eating lots of wheat-bran only cereals. Fibre taken as part of whole food isn't a problem.
- Vitamin A deficiency causes low oestrogen. You can get levels up by eating more betacarotene in orange, yellow and green vegetables or fruits. (Taking vitamin A supplements is not safe long term and at high doses.)
- Antibiotics reduce substantial numbers of the gut bacteria needed to convert oestrogen into a more active form for use in the body. Yoghurt and cultured milks can eventually improve bowel colonies, but it's better to avoid antibiotics, except in severe infection.
- Overexercising reduces the levels of circulating oestrogens, and can cause stopped periods and low bone density.
- Smoking alters the metabolism of oestrogen so that more of the inactive oestrogen is produced. If you smoke, you'll be relatively oestrogen deficient, and have an earlier menopause and an increased risk of bone fractures.
- Some drugs, ones called GnRH agonists, are used to create a menopause-like state to try to control endometriosis and will cause the usual side effects of menopause as well.

Treatment

If a doctor perceives there is a problem, the Pill or hormone replacement therapy (HRT) will probably be prescribed. A natural therapy or self care approach would follow the obvious path suggested by possible causes listed above, like not overexercising or getting too thin, eating a moderate fibre intake, avoiding cigarettes and antibiotics, and making sure you don't have a vitamin A deficiency. Also eat food from plants which contain oestrogens (listed in the section on plant oestrogens in the Self Care chapter), and also foods containing steroidal saponins. Substances called saponins in foods and herbs seem to improve mineral uptake, and can lower blood cholesterol levels. Foods with saponins include soya products, all legumes and potatoes with their skins on. You may be prescribed herbs containing high levels of steroidal saponins, including *Chamaelirium luteum*, *Trillium erectum*, *Dioscorea villosa* and *Aletris farinosa*. Some of these seem to have definite oestrogen-like and hormone balancing effects.

DIAGNOSIS

Common tests

There are a few ways to tell whether menopause is approaching. Single tests are not all that reliable and are generally added to any symptoms you're getting to make a diagnosis. Sometimes the symptoms are the best indicators anyway.

Blood tests for levels of FSH are not infallible, but are often used to diagnose menopause. High levels of FSH indicate declining levels of oestrogen. FSH levels often fluctuate around the menopause and can give misleading results. The FSH levels will remain consistently high once you have become menopausal, but by then you won't need a blood test to tell you.

Sometimes the blood levels of oestrogen and progesterone are measured to see whether they are within the normal limits, but this is an even more unreliable test than the FSH level and in most cases a waste of time and money.

The vaginal walls can show early changes which are caused by the declining oestrogen levels. When examined by a doctor, they might look thinner and drier, and sometimes bleed. These signs are generally quite late, but you might develop them early if you have symptoms of chronically low oestrogen (low body weight, a strenuous exercise regime, or a very high-fibre diet).

A menstrual diary in which you also record other symptoms will be a great help.

Often doctors will prescribe HRT on the basis of symptoms even if blood tests are normal. If the symptoms improve, they are assumed to be related to the menopause. Natural therapists will also prescribe on the basis of symptoms and will usually try to regulate hormone levels and establish normal period patterns.

PERIOD SYMPTOMS DIARY: Record the relevant coded number to describe your bleeding and symptoms.

BLEEDING: 0—none 1—slight 2—moderate 3—heavy 4—heavy and clots
SYMPTOMS: 0—none 1—mild; does not interfere with activities 2—moderate; interferes with activities 3—severe; disabling; unable to function

Day of cycle	1	2	3	4	5	6	7	8	9	10	11	12	13	14	15	16	17	18	19	20	21	22	23	24	25	26	27	28	29	30	31	32	33	34	35	36
DATE																																				
BLEEDING																																				
PMS-A SYMPTOMS:																																				
Nervous tension																																				
Mood swings																																				
Irritability																																				
Anxiety																																				
PMS-H SYMPTOMS:																																				
Weight gain																																				
Swelling of extremities																																				
Breast tenderness																																				
Abdominal bloating																																				
PMS-C SYMPTOMS:																																				
Headache																																				
Craving for sweets																																				
Increased appetite																																				
Heart pounding																																				
Fatigue																																				
Dizziness or faintness																																				
PMS-D SYMPTOMS:																																				
Depression																																				
Forgetfulness																																				
Crying																																				
Confusion																																				
Insomnia																																				
PMS-P SYMPTOMS:																																				
Pain																																				
Cramps																																				
Backache																																				
General aches/pain																																				

You can photocopy this diary to use indefinitely.

WHEN TO SEE A DOCTOR

Even if you're coping fine with menopausal symptoms and don't think you need any help, you need to see a doctor if you have:

- any vaginal bleeding, no matter how slight, coming a year or more after the last period
- mid-cycle bleeding or bleeding between periods no matter how light
- bleeding after sex
- persistently heavy periods
- any unusual spotting or bleeding which worries you
- unexpected pain associated with periods or bleeding.

Managing the Symptoms

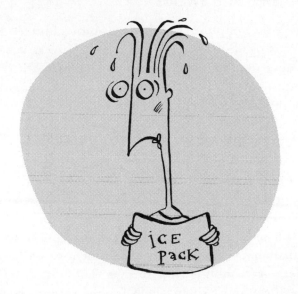

ERRATIC PERIODS AND THE ENDOMETRIUM

If ovulation becomes erratic, the cycle length and regularity of the period will have an effect on the endometrium (cells lining the uterus). The endometrium tends to be exposed to lower levels of oestrogen for longer periods of time, and to be exposed to little or no progesterone (which is only produced once you've ovulated).

As a result, the endometrium tends to bleed more easily, and periods can become really heavy. Spotting is common and in rare cases, the endometrial cells can undergo pre-cancerous or even cancerous changes because of the effects of oestrogen.

HOT FLUSHES AND SWEATS

These are the symptoms which most women find the most 'embarrassing'. Sitting in the middle of a business meeting or arguing over the washing machine repair bill, some women are given a horrible reminder of uncontrollable adolescent blushing. Some of the modern rewriting of menopause suggests that women just call them 'power surges'. Although most of us are more likely to think, 'Bugger power surges for a joke. I'm not an electrical sub-station, I just want my body to behave itself.'

About three-quarters of all menopausal women experience some form of hot flushes; and about one-third of them will seek treatment. Two Australian studies indicated that almost 40 per cent of the menopausal women experienced 'troubling' hot flushes, but not all women took medication or sought help for their symptoms.

Flushes are likely to be as different as the women who have them. Some have fleeting hot and sweaty feelings; others might be drenched with sweat, feel uncomfortably hot, go red in the face and/or have heart palpitations. Sometimes hot flushes come with headaches, a sense of increased pressure in the head, vagueness, transient chills, fatigue, dizziness or nausea.

The body usually adjusts to the changing hormones

after about a year and the hot flushes disappear completely. In very rare cases they will last for five to ten years after the period has stopped.

Flushes are caused by oestrogen decline, and a surge of luteinising hormone (LH). Hot flushes are more severe if you are very thin, probably because body fat helps to make extra oestrogen. Women who become menopausal suddenly, or at a younger age than usual, often experience severe hot flushes. Maybe the body's not prepared for the sudden loss of oestrogen.

After a flush there is often a slight drop in temperature caused by loss of body heat from sweating. Temperature fluctuations can cause the on-again, off-again problem with clothes (so that's why older women start wearing cardigans!) and lead to a serious disturbance in sleep patterns—thrashing about, in other words.

Lately, there has been speculation that hot flushes are not just a nuisance and that they may serve a positive role. One theory is that the increase in body temperature sets the stage for a healthier old age by burning up toxins and stimulating the immune response (similar to the increase in immune activity when we have a temperature caused by a cold or the flu). Another is that they represent surges of creative and positive energy. You little sub-station, you.

The medical approach

The medical treatment of any menopausal symptom is almost always hormone replacement therapy (HRT)—and hot flushes respond well to this medication. Somewhere between 60 and 90 per cent of women with hot flushes who are treated with HRT improve dramatically. In view of the lack of information on the long-term effects of HRT, natural remedies may be more appropriate unless there are compelling reasons why HRT should be considered.

Natural therapies

Natural remedies are prescribed after taking into account all the factors that might contribute to the menopausal symptoms—including lifestyle and medical elements. The need to differentiate between the differing triggers for hot flushes has long been accepted in herbal medicine. It makes the treatment more complex, but much more likely to bring relief of the symptom *and* the cause. It also means that no one medicine will help all women with hot flushes and prescriptions need to be tailored to the individual.

Herbs

Herbs containing plant oestrogens have been used for centuries for the management of hot flushes and other oestrogen-related symptoms. Like all herbs referred to in this book, they must be prescribed by a trained herbalist. All plant oestrogens are many times weaker than synthetic, laboratory-made oestrogens or the oestrogens made in the body. But a menopausal woman produces very little oestrogen of her own, so the plant oestrogens become more dominant, and can do some good.

Of particular interest to herbalists is *Cimicifuga racemosa*, long recognised and used in the European, American, Indian and Chinese traditions for menopausal symptoms. It has been the subject of a number of open and blind trials in Germany where many medical doctors routinely prescribe it for menopausal symptoms. The results are very good, especially for hot flushes and vaginal dryness.

Anxiety
Anxiety or worry can bring on hot flushes, and a number of herbs can be useful. They include *Hypericum perforatum*, for flushes associated with anxiety depression states; *Humulus lupulus* (hops), for flushing and insomnia; *Tilia cordata* (lime or linden flowers) and *Leonurus cardiaca* (motherwort) for menopausal symptoms which are accompanied by palpitations; and *Verbena officinalis* (vervain) for anxiety associated with thyroid dysfunction.

Fatigue and overwork
The herbal adaptogens most commonly used are *Panax ginseng*, *Eleuthrococcus senticosus*, *Codonopsis pilosa*, *Glycyrrhiza glabra* and *Astragalus membranaceus*. They help the body 'adapt' to the effects of stress and fatigue and as a 'side effect', reduce the severity of flushing.

Night sweats
Humulus lupulus (hops) contains oestrogen-like substances and is good for night sweats and insomnia. In some cases, simply improving the quality of sleep with herbal hypnotics will put a lid on hot flushes. *Valeriana officinalis*, *Scutellaria laterifolia*, *Passiflora incarnate*, *Avena sativa* and *Matricaria recutita* are commonly available either as teas or in tablets.

27

Severe sweating

The two herbs which are useful for menopausal sweating are *Salvia officinalis* and *Astragalus membranaceus*, and they are usually combined with other remedies for flushing. One common Chinese formula for sweating associated with weakness contains *Astragalus membranaceus*, *Codonopsis pilosa*, *Angelica sinensis*, *Cimicifuga racemosa*, *Atractylodes macrocephala* and *Bupleurum falcatum*. *Salvia officinalis* (garden sage) is mildly 'oestrogenic' and improves circulation to the brain.

Supplements

Vitamin E

Studies in the 1950s showed vitamin E is useful for menopausal symptoms. In clinical trials, doses ranged from 10 to 100 milligrams a day (100 IU is equivalent to 67 milligrams). Vitamin E reduces the severity of hot flushes and other symptoms associated with menopause. Between 100 and 500 IU a day is the usual dose. (Women with blood pressure or heart problems should get advice from their health care practitioner before using vitamin E.)

Vitamin C and the bioflavonoids

In the early 1960s, the bioflavonoid hesperidin, derived from citrus fruits, was shown to reduce the severity of hot flushes, but more research is needed to know why. Sometimes moderate to high doses of vitamin C seem to help too, maybe by increasing the viability of oestrogens in the body.

Evening primrose oil

Many women find that evening primrose oil is useful for a variety of menopausal symptoms, including flushing, mood changes and fluid retention. The dose range to try is between 1 and 3 grams daily, but studies have shown it's not much better than a placebo. If symptoms improve with evening primrose oil then you probably had PMS rather than menopausal problems. Evening primrose oil is also rather expensive and the other herbs and supplements are often more cost-effective for menopausal women. Diet can also be altered to take in more essential fatty acids. (See Good Fats and Bad Fats in the 20 Diet Hints in the Self Care chapter.)

Self care

- Dress to reduce the severity of the symptoms. It is most useful to wear a bikini under a fake fur coat. Oh, alright. Try light and loose-fitting clothing from natural fibre, such as cotton; it's much less likely to aggravate sweating. Try a lighter layer underneath a jacket or cardigan you can shrug off, and cotton night gear, and you can sleep on a towel or folded sheet which you can throw out of the bed if it gets wet, rather than having to change the sheets.

- Avoid food and drink that seems to aggravate hot flushes. Culprits include coffee, excessively spicy foods and alcohol. Drinking or eating foods that are extremely hot can also trigger a flush, and simply eating foods at a lower temperature can help. If you love going out for a curry and a few drinks, get ready to hurl your cardie on and off all night.

- Here's a simple home remedy for the treatment of hot flushes and sweating: Chop about six fresh sage leaves and soak overnight in the juice of a lemon. In the morning, strain and drink the juice diluted with water to taste. Two weeks of this mixture will usually control flushing and sweating, and also improves digestion and concentration. It should not be continued for longer than two weeks. You can have another round of it after two months.
- Eat 'plant oestrogens'. Eating just 100 grams of tofu and 2 dessertspoons of freshly ground linseeds (use a clean coffee grinder) every day can reduce hot flushes and vaginal dryness. Researchers have also seen a link between eating foods with high levels of plant oestrogens and lower rates of oestrogen- dependent cancers. (More info on the plant oestrogens is in the Self Care chapter.)

DRYNESS

Declining oestrogen levels can dry out the tissues of the vagina, vulva and urethra, and the eyes and mouth. About 40 per cent of women over 55 have some dryness and about half of these report moderate to severe symptoms. The severity seems to be connected to dietary factors, body weight and stress. Like other menopausal symptoms, there is a large variation in symptoms. A range of problems might be experienced, from none at all, to varying degrees of burning, dryness and irritation. Vaginal, vulval and urinary tract symptoms can play havoc with your sex life and general comfort.

Vaginal dryness, thinning of the vaginal walls and urinary symptoms usually happen after menopause, but sometimes happen before it. Vaginal dryness during sex can cause mild discomfort through to pain. Less oestrogen can also lead to increased alkalinity of the vagina which can cause irritation, itching or infections. Eating more yoghurt, or even applying it, can help.

When urethral tissue is affected by declining oestrogens, recurring problems can include weeing all the time, a burning sensation, cystitis, and incontinence. These complaints require active treatment, and all women who develop urinary tract symptoms around the menopause, or later, should consider mucous membrane change as a potential cause: only treating the urinary tract infection will almost certainly mean it will keep coming back.

The medical approach

Vaginal dryness, soreness, and painful sex can be treated with HRT or oestrogen-containing creams, tablets or pessaries. They should be used at night. These are explained in full detail on page 56 in the HRT chapter.

Collagen disorders which affect other tissues such as bones, the pelvic organs and the skin, are increasingly being treated with oestrogen pills. And doctors will usually prescribe HRT.

Natural therapies

Natural therapists recommend creams for vaginal dryness. An aqueous cream (like plain old sorbolene) or vitamin E cream from the chemist can be used as a base to which herbs and oils are added. This can be made at home: 10

millilitres of infused oil of *Calendula officinalis* (marigold); 30 millilitres of olive oil; 20 millilitres of the oil of evening primrose in 75 grams of aqueous cream. Apply two or three times daily to the vulva and inside the vagina. If you make a large batch, store it in the fridge.

Oestrogenic herbs can also be used in creams, since oestrogen is well absorbed through the skin. Middle Eastern women reportedly use a poultice of *Trigonella foenum-graecum* (fenugreek), but the pungent odour makes it rather antisocial and would probably put you off your curry. Using a water-based lubricant, such as 'Wet Stuff' or KY jelly during sex will also help. It's available from ordinary old chemists and supermarkets or those shops which sell mysterious battery-operated items and black leather French maid's uniforms with optional thonging.

Self care
Eat plant oestrogens, especially linseeds (see under Plant Oestrogens in the Self Care chapter for more info).

'PMS'-TYPE SYMPTOMS

Women in their forties with PMS symptoms are often told or believe that they are 'menopausal'. Symptoms related to hormone fluctuations are not necessarily menopausal unless you also have irregular periods—and even then there may be other causes. Some of the 'menopausal symptoms' like hot flushes, migraines and palpitations are experienced by women in their twenties and thirties—not to mention men—who are not menopausal, and who are not automatically prescribed HRT.

One study of recently menopausal women showed that although hot flushes increased when periods stopped, symptoms like sore breasts, irritability, excitability, depression and poor concentration improved after the period, which suggests that these symptoms are more likely to be related to periods than to the menopause.

Evening primrose oil capsules are commonly recommended or self-prescribed for these symptoms, even though they are no better than placebo for true menopausal symptoms when scientifically trialled. Evening primrose is, however, useful for PMS, and so if you feel better on the capsules you've probably got PMS symptoms rather than menopausal ones.

So, if you are 40-something with fairly regular periods and no hot flushes or vaginal dryness, don't just assume a problem is caused by oncoming menopause. You might respond better to remedies for PMS. There is a sister book to this one called *Problem Periods* which deals specifically with period related problems if you need more information on PMS or irregular bleeding around menopause.

MOOD CHANGES

About one in ten women experience depression, anxiety or feelings of inadequacy around menopause, but there is some dispute about why it happens. Some researchers have shown that these symptoms are related to hormone changes, others found these symptoms were more common when women had pre-existing problems such as depression, difficulties with coping generally, or PMS. We could call these the 'I don't want to go through menopause' theory and the 'hormone theory'.

According to the 'I don't want to go through menopause' theory, women with a negative attitude to menopause, or life in general, were much more likely to experience problems. This theory says that any mood changes are caused by attitude, not hormones.

The 'hormone theory' reckons that stress caused by mood changes may lower oestrogen levels and aggravate menopausal symptoms, which then causes more stress. In one study, menopausal women recovering from depression had higher levels of oestrogen as they improved. Sleep deprivation due to hot flushes is believed to be another cause of depression. When oestrogen levels are increased, sleep patterns return to normal.

Treatment for mood swings is varied because the causes are often diverse. You might be depressed before your period because of hormones, or you might be depressed before your period because the bank manager keeps shouting at you. When PMS is the cause, symptoms will happen before the period. Whatever the choice of treatment—vitamin, herb, drug, or counselling—it is far better that the cause of the depression or mood swings be found rather than prescribing something to lift the mood temporarily.

The Medical Approach
Some doctors commonly prescribe HRT, believing that it alleviates the mood changes associated with menopause.

 34

It doesn't, however, appear to be any better than a placebo in having an effect on mood. It does improve flushing and vaginal symptoms though, and this might cheer you up.

Anti-depressant drugs or sedatives should rarely be needed, not least because so many people have become dependent on them and they don't go to the root of the problem. Doctors may also suggest counselling.

Natural therapies

Hypericum performatum, a herb which has been compared to tricyclic anti-depressants in effects, has a long history of use for menopausal complaints which are associated with anxiety or depression. Herbalists refer to this plant as a nervine, specific to the management of menopausal complaints. Again, make sure you get to the cause of the problem and don't just take an anti-depressant, herbal or otherwise.

Tired women often think that their symptoms must be due to menopause. In reality, they may be due to any of the usual causes of fatigue including hypoglycaemia, iron deficiency, adrenal exhaustion, too much exercise or depression. A series of blood tests may be needed to tell what's wrong. Women who are well, but tired all the time, respond to combinations of the appropriate herbs for the nervous system, adaptogens and vitamin B complex, along with appropriate dietary changes and increase in exercise. *Eleuthrococcus senticosus* (Siberian ginseng) at doses of 500 milligrams to 1 gram twice a day combined with a standard vitamin B complex tablet twice daily, is often effective.

Self care

For all types of mood changes, simple lifestyle changes, such as exercise, stress management techniques, yoga, and meditation are helpful. Walking daily for half an hour has been shown to improve mood. Often depression, anxiety or self-esteem problems will improve with seeing a good counsellor. B vitamins, particularly vitamin B6, or any other remedies used for PMS are helpful for mood changes.

MIGRAINES

Premenstrual migraines can get worse approaching menopause. The headaches are often thought to be caused by blood sugar fluctuations, and the rapid decline in oestrogens just before a period. The oestrogen freefall can trigger a blood vessel spasm, which causes the headache. Treatment for premenstrual migraines is almost always in conjunction with the prescription herb *Cimicifuga racemosa* (black cohosh) which can help symptoms of fluctuating oestrogen levels. Increasing the amount of plant oestrogens in the diet can also help.

Healthy Bones after Menopause

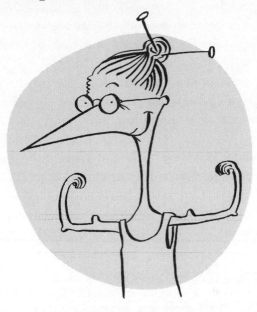

Bone density and osteoporosis are some of the big buzz-words in menopause. Basically, osteoporosis is a disorder characterised by low bone density, leading to a greater risk of bone fractures. In very severe cases, curvature of the spine (the rudely titled 'dowager's hump') and severely restricted movement can result. Bone density refers to the amount of minerals in your bone, not how large bones are. It's usually measured by the amount of mineral per unit area of the bone. For bones to remain healthy and resistant to fracture, it makes sense to keep your bone density high. This isn't a magic process in which you can just take a pill.

Exercise patterns and diet can result in fluctuations in bone density all through your life. The main reason why low bone density becomes such a big issue for women in later life is because women's bones are made stronger by oestrogen, and your ovaries stop making it after the menopause.

Menopause is late to start doing something about protecting your bones, but in most cases it's not too late. Bone is constantly remodelling itself and interacting in a wide range of natural biochemical events. It is a dynamic, growing tissue. If it wasn't, fractures wouldn't heal. Bone cell activity can be speeded up or slowed down by changes in mineral intake, hormone levels and exercise patterns. These factors, especially as hormone levels change, can be complex.

RISK FACTORS FOR OSTEOPOROSIS

The big risk factors for losing bone density are not enough oestrogen, not enough nutrition, not enough calcium, and not enough exercise, but not necessarily in that order.

Physical characteristics: Being a fair-skinned, small-framed woman with a relative who's had osteoporosis increases your statistical chance of developing weak bones. (Men have a higher initial peak bone mass and don't have the rapid loss seen in women in the early postmenopausal years.) Shamefully, it appears at the time of writing that there are no statistics available on the osteoporosis risk to Aboriginal women.

Repeated weight loss diets, poor or fad diets: Restricted diets result in low body weight, lead to a reduction in bone density. Dieters, ballet dancers and athletes who maintain or maintained unusually low body fat levels are all at high risk, especially if the periods stop as well.

High protein diets: Excess protein intake increases calcium excretion in the urine. The calcium loss may persist for several months after dietary re-adjustment. This is particularly significant for those on repeated short-term or long-term 'low/no carbohydrate', high protein diets.

Caffeine and alcohol: Alcohol and caffeine increase the rate at which minerals are lost from bone and excreted in the urine.

Sugar and salt: Both sugar and salt eaten to excess increase loss of bone minerals and increase loss via the urine.

High fibre: Women with excessively high fibre intakes have lower oestrogen levels and bone density than other women. Phytates in grains can form an insoluble bond with the essential minerals and reduce absorption. This is not much of a problem in Australia as most women don't have enough fibre rather than too much.

Sedentary lifestyle: Not exercising increases mineral loss from bone. Calcium is even lost from bone during a normal night's sleep. Exercise that increases bone strength is usually described as 'weight bearing'—for example walking rather than swimming or bike-riding in which the body is supported.

Prolonged bed rest: Bed rest increases mineral excretion in the urine because bones are not subject to the usual weight-bearing stress.

Smoking: Smoking decreases oestrogen production and increases oestrogen breakdown. Post-menopausal women who smoke fracture bones more often than non-smokers. Women who are on HRT and smoke may have up to 50 per cent less oestrogen than non-smokers.

Other contributing possibilities include

Malabsorption syndromes, chronic diarrhoea: Complaints which reduce mineral uptake from the gut can adversely affect bone density. These include coeliac disease, Crohn's disease, ulcerative colitis and fat absorption problems.

Premature menopause: Low oestrogen levels at an earlier age reduces the retention of calcium in bone. The number of years since menopause is a better indicator of bone density than age.

No periods (doctors call it amenorrhoea): Rigorous exercise, too much dieting, anorexia nervosa, or hormone imbalances are associated with low levels of oestrogen and can lead to a loss of bone mass.

Other illnesses: Diabetes, hyperparathyroidism, rheumatoid arthritis, alcoholism, epilepsy (because of drugs), scurvy, Cushing's syndrome, thyrotoxicosis, the surgical removal of any part of the stomach and inherited disorders of the connective tissue are associated with an increased risk of osteoporosis.

Drugs, etc.: You should check with your doctor or pharmacist about the effect on calcium levels of any drug you are prescribed or buy over the counter. Some common drugs that we know decrease calcium and have a negative impact on bone density include cortisone, diuretics, anti-convulsants such as Dilantin, anti-coagulants such as Heparin, thyroxine and some antibiotics including tetracyclines. Aluminium can decrease bone density. Aluminium is regularly added to buffered aspirin, antacids, toothpastes, baking powders, cooking utensils, dental amalgams, cigarette filters, food additives, aluminium foil and cosmetics. Be especially careful of aluminium cookwear and aluminium foil if you are cooking acidic foods like tomatoes, acid fruits and fish with lemon wrapped in foil. Food acids release aluminium into your food and substantially increase your intake. Fluoride decreases the rate of vertebral fracture, but may increase the incidence of hip fracture. Long-term, low-dose exposure to fluoride in drinking water has been associated with lower bone density.

MEASURING THE PROBLEM

If you fall into a significant risk category of osteoporosis it's a good idea to have a bone density measurement test. Your doctor can arrange a test for you.

Dual Energy X-ray Absorptiometry (DEXA): This X-Ray method is very precise and can measure small changes in the bone density of the hip and spine. A very low level of radiation exposure is used.

Single Photon Absorptiometry (SPA): This method is less expensive than the DEXA, but it has the disadvantage of measuring the bone density of only the forearm, which may not accurately reflect the bone density of the hip or spine. The radiation exposure is double that of the DEXA, but is still small, at about ten times less than an average X-ray.

'Plain' X-rays: An X-ray will detect osteoporosis once the amount of bone mineral loss is 30 per cent or more of the total bone mass. This makes plain X-rays unsuitable for evaluation of bone density because you can only see a problem once it's already very advanced.

Computerised Tomography (CT or CAT scan): A CAT scan is used to detect bone mineral loss in the spinal region. It is not used to detect general bone density loss or to monitor changes in bone density.

BUILDING BETTER BONES

To stay on the right course to have healthy, strong bones, there are three key issues:

- adequate intake of the correct nutrients;
- proper absorption of these nutrients from (ahem, this is a technical term) gut;
- satisfactory retention of nutrients in bone.

Improvement in all of the three areas tends to lead to cumulative results, and so it's good to work on all these things while pursuing some kind of useful exercise program. Your doctor or natural therapist can help tailor-make one for you.

Intake

A balanced diet (see the Self Care chapter) is essential for bone health. This diet should include a high proportion of vegetables, grains and beans, some dairy products and fruit in moderation. A vegetarian diet after the age of 50 improves bone density because protein intake is lower and calcium loss is reduced.

The major bone minerals

Calcium and magnesium are the Big Two bone minerals, and we go into detail about them and their recommended daily allowances in the Minerals section of the Self Care chapter. For the whole lowdown on calcium see from page 114 and for magnesium from page 123.

Retaining nutrients in bone

Exercise: The effects of calcium, oestrogen and exercise tend to be cumulative. Even though there is more benefit gained from exercise up until menopause, an exercise-related increase in bone density is seen after menopause, as well. Any exercise, but particularly types which make the large muscles work, has the potential to improve bone mass. The best type is weight-bearing exercise like walking, running or playing sport.

Resistance strength training (like weights) also improves bone density in women before and after menopause. In addition, resistance exercise increases muscle mass, which is another casualty of being menopausal. Post-menopausal women can lose up to one-third of their total muscle mass by the time they are 80 unless they continue to exercise, meaning they are weaker, less agile and more likely to injure themselves or break bones. Swimming and cycling are also important even though they are not classically included in the weight-bearing group.

Exercise should be daily or every second day for 60 minutes for maximum benefits. Needless to say, consult a trainer or book to decide what's good for you and speak to your doctor first.

Body weight

Body weight has two main effects on bone mass: the weight-bearing stimulus to bone formation is greater in heavier women, and throughout life women make a percentage of their oestrogens from fatty tissue. This may be one of the reasons why plumper women tend to have fewer symptoms of oestrogen decline at menopause, such as hot flushes and vaginal dryness.

Hormone Replacement Therapy (HRT)

HRT is an effective medication in the prevention and treatment of osteoporosis, and substantially slows post-menopausal bone loss. Exercise and complete dietary supplements, although not as potent, should be considered as the first line of intervention in maintaining bone health. They improve so many other areas of health, such as general fitness, nutritional status and lower stress levels.

TREATING LOW BONE DENSITY AND OSTEOPOROSIS

Women with osteoporosis can adopt all of the strategies outlined for maintaining healthy bones, but with a little more enthusiasm, to treat low bone density. Someone with specific experience should supervise exercise regimes for women with osteoporosis so that good techniques improve bone density and muscle strength while preventing injury or useless activity.

HRT is still the best drug available to improve bone density. Positive effects, such as the fracture risk decreasing by 30–50 per cent, are seen with all types of oestrogen and oestrogen-with-progestogen HRT, including tablets, patches, gels and implants. Vaginal creams and pessaries can be expected to have negligible effects. Bio-identical HRT should also be useful, but research is lacking.

However the issues surrounding HRT are complex and becoming increasingly so. Fracture risk increases and bone density starts to drop within a year of stopping HRT and it needs to be taken for many years, if not life-long, to protect bones. Herein lies a problem. Both breast and ovarian cancer risk increase with long-term HRT use, and although these risks are comparatively small, whether to take HRT is a challenging decision for an individual woman. Also, heart and blood clotting problems can increase. Read the sections on HRT, and HRT and Your Heart for more info.

Fortunately there are other choices. Evista and Livial are oestrogen-like drugs that do not increase breast cancer risk, although, like HRT, they are a problem for the heart. Fosamax (a bisphosphonate) is used to improve calcium levels in bone. It is available as a once-a-week tablet which reduces risk of oesophageal irritation. Fosamax must be taken while standing up and away from calcium supplements and food. Calcitrol and cholecalciferol are Vitamin D-like substances that are also worth considering.

Your Heart

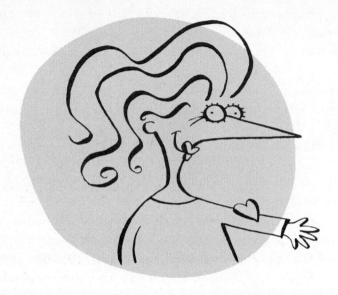

If you want to lower your post-menopause risk of cardio-vascular (heart) disease, having a heart attack, a stroke or developing hardened arteries, there's a lot you can do. For example, stop having fried camembert sandwiches for breakfast.

Some risk factors, like age, sex, and family history, can't be changed, and women with inherited blood fat disorders may need to take drugs to lower their choles-terol levels if their healthy change of diet hasn't helped. HRT, once thought to be the answer for women with high risk of cardiovascular disease, is now known to actually increase the risk if it's taken by women with established heart disease. It also increases the tendency to blood clot formation, especially in the first year. An increase in blood triglyceride levels (a type of blood fat) has also been observed when women take HRT. Many women will not consider HRT worth the risk.

RISK FACTORS FOR HEART DISEASE

Fags: We don't want to create any unnecessary panic BUT IF YOU DON'T STOP THAT RIGHT NOW YOU COULD DIEEEEEEEE. Smoking substantially increases the risk of all serious heart problems, including it stopping altogether. Australian women aged 35 to 69 years who smoke are 3.5 times more likely to suffer from a first-time heart attack than non-smoking women of the same age; and the risk of sudden death increases by two to four times. Heavy smokers increase their risk of heart disease by up to five times that of non-smokers, and the risk is increased still further if other risk factors are present, especially high blood pressure and high cholesterol.

The risk of stroke is increased in smokers. The more you smoke, or the longer you do, the bigger your risks. The incidence of many other heart and blood flow problems are massively increased in smokers. Passive smoking carries a 30 per cent increased risk of heart disease. The sooner you stop, the sooner your risk level starts to change.

Blood pressure: High blood pressure, also called hypertension, affects around 6.3 per cent of women and may elevate risk of heart disease by up to four times.

Obesity: Obesity, or too much body fat, can be measured by using the body mass index (BMI). You can calculate your BMI, as seen previously on page 17, by using the equation below. The National Health and Medical Research Council has defined 'acceptable' weight as a BMI of 20.0 to 25.0, 'overweight' as a BMI of over 25 up to 30.0, and 'obese' as a BMI of over 30.0. (Incidentally, a BMI can only be accurate on a person who has completely finished puberty so you're probably safe there.)

To calculate your BMI, your weight in kilograms is divided by the square of your height in metres. For example, if you are 70 kg and 1.65 m in height, your BMI is calculated this way: $70 \div (1.65 \times 1.65) = 25.7$.

Long-term studies tend to show a relationship between obesity and cardiovascular disease, but this is not true of all studies. In fact, it may be the other conditions which often occur with obesity, such as poor physical fitness, high blood pressure and high blood cholesterol, that are responsible for the increased risk of heart and blood vessel disease.

It may not be an individual's actual weight at all, but more where the weight is. This is called the 'body fat distribution'. When weight is distributed mainly around the abdomen (apple-shaped), the risk of cardiovascular disease is greater, and some studies show an even stronger relationship between abdominal obesity and heart disease than BMI. Remember too that muscle weighs more than fat.

Booze: The National Health and Medical Research Council warns women not to regularly have more than two to four standard drinks a day, and presumably their office parties are a little dull. As little as two drinks or more a day can be enough to progressively increase blood pressure, and can lead to an increased death rate from heart disease. However, a low alcohol intake (up to two drinks of wine, for example) may reduce the risk of heart disease because of the presence of tannins which are strong anti-oxidants and are cardio-protective. Bottom line: go easy.

High blood cholesterol: You can get a blood cholesterol level test from your health practitioner. The National Heart Foundation defines high cholesterol as being higher than 5.5 millimols per litre in an adult. High blood cholesterol is linked to the development and progression of hardened arteries to heart disease. Perhaps more importantly, it is the blood levels of LDL (low density lipoprotein) 'bad' cholesterol that are proportional to the risk of heart disease, whilst HDL (high density lipoprotein) 'good' cholesterol tends to be protective. Ask your health practitioner for more details.

Elevated cholesterol has a tendency to oxidise (go rancid) in the blood and this is another serious risk factor for developing heart and blood vessel disease (such as stroke and blood clots). Eating plenty of anti-oxidant-rich foods such as green, orange and red vegetables, green tea, onions and garlic will help to reduce this risk. Eating Hot Buttered Lardy Meaty Egg Surprise will increase your cholesterol levels.

Diabetes: Diabetes mellitus is associated with changes in fat metabolism and abnormal blood lipids (high blood lipids, high LDL and low HDL). This leads to an increased incidence of hardened arteries and cardiovascular diseases. Your health practitioner can help you with guarding against this where possible.

Lying around: The more you sit on your bot-bot watching the telly instead of dancing, walking or having wild sex (exercising), the higher your risk of developing cardiovascular diseases. For example, those in sedentary occupations are twice as likely to die from heart disease than those in active occupations.

HOW TO PROTECT YOUR HEART

Exercise: It needs to be regular and to increase heart rate. This can be achieved by fast walking, jogging, dancing, or aerobics. There should be a component that will help make you more flexible. Stretching or yoga classes are ideal. Some attempt should be made to increase muscle strength, such as gym work, or lifting weights at home.

Diet: Diets high in saturated fats encourage high LDL ('bad' cholesterol), but low HDL ('good' cholesterol) levels and are associated with an increased risk of cardiovascular disease. Diets that are lower in animal fat (except Omega-3 fats) and refined carbohydrates, help to reduce body fat and the waist to hip ratio. Being overweight and having an apple-shaped rather than pear-shaped body are both associated with heart disease.

New research has shown that phyto-oestrogens, particularly the consumption of soy products, reduces cholesterol levels and blood pressure levels. These findings, combined with the evidence on breast cancer rates from cultures where people eat plenty of soy, suggests soy could reduce your cancer risk, improve bone density, reduce symptoms associated with menopause as well as protect your heart.

A low-fat diet with an increased intake of oily fish, anti-oxidants, fibre, phyto-oestrogens and complex carbohydrates is recommended. Women with high cholesterol levels should avoid saturated (animal) fats, but include oily fish, olive and seed oils. This diet is outlined on page 103, and information on good and bad fats is in the 20 Diet Hints section of the Self Care chapter.

HRT AND YOUR HEART

HRT reduces cholesterol and protects blood vessels, but increases blood clot formation, and risk of heart attacks and strokes. This is why women were initially told to take HRT to *prevent* or *treat* heart disease and blood clots, and latertold that it was unwise to do either of these things—the expected benefits just didn't materialise.

Recent studies have shown that women with heart disease get worse if they take HRT, and that healthy women on HRT experience more adverse events than those not on it. One research paper released in July 2002 showed that combined HRT (oestrogen with progesterone) increased blood clots by 100 per cent, strokes by 41 per cent, and heart attacks by 29 per cent. Evista and Livial are no help either. Stay away from all of them if you have a heart or clotting problem. And take care if you're travelling, as the risk of blood clots (deep vein thrombosis) may also increase on long plane trips.

Hormone Replacement Therapy (HRT)

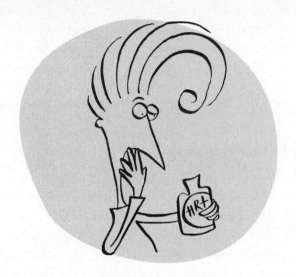

Hormone Replacement Therapy (HRT) is no longer recommended for long-term use by healthy women to prevent heart disease and osteoporosis. This is since the release of two studies in July 2002 showing 'continuous' oestrogen and progestogen caused more harm than good and finding that oestrogen alone increased risk of ovarian cancer with long-term use. A hoped-for benefit in reducing risk of Alzheimer's or improving cognitive function has also not eventuated, and preventative HRT for these disorders is not appropriate.

HRT is considered safe short-term (12 months or less) for the treatment of menopausal symptoms such as hot flushes. It is still recommended long-term to treat established osteoporosis, but any woman who has been on or is considering going on HRT long-term should do so only after assessment of her individual situation.

This section looks at the types of HRT and explains their risks and benefits. Newer treatments to reduce the adverse consequences of menopause, Evista and Livial, are also under scrutiny. You should also read about your chances of developing heart complaints (pages 47–50), osteoporosis (pages 38–41) and breast cancer (pages 62–3) to help you decide whether to take HRT or not—or you could identify risks and try to do something positive about them—exercising more, for example so that you won't need to even consider HRT.

TYPES OF HRT

Oestrogen only
Only women who have had a hysterectomy can use oestrogen alone—women with a uterus need progesterone as well to protect the uterine lining.

Tablets
Oestrogen is recommended for menopausal symptoms such as hot flushes and may be suggested to prevent or treat osteoporosis. Common brands are Premarin, Ogen, Ovestin, Estrofem, Zumenon, Genoral and Progynova.

Research has shown that long-term use of oestrogen alone increases risk of ovarian and breast cancer, as well as heart attacks, strokes and the formation of blood clots.

Patches and gels
Patches include Climara, Dermestril, Estraderm, Femtran and Menorest. An oestrogen-impregnated, adhesive patch is applied to the skin, usually the buttock, through which oestrogen is easily absorbed into the body. Sandrena gel contains oestrogen and is rubbed onto the skin daily. Oestrogen patches and gels may have much the same risks and benefits as oestrogen tablets, but are much less likely to cause nausea or liver and gall bladder problems (oestrogen goes to the liver first when it is taken orally).

Implants
Implants are small 'tablets' that are injected under the skin. The oestrogen is slowly absorbed into the blood stream and the implant is replaced every four to eight months or when symptoms return. Risks and benefits are pretty much the same as for tablets. Oral progestogens are prescribed for women with a uterus. Some implants also contain testosterone and are used to combat low sex drive.

Vaginal creams or pessaries
Creams (Ovestin and Premarin) and pessaries (Ovestin Ovula or Vagifem) are a better choice than tablets or patches to relieve vaginal dryness and urinary symptoms such as burning and irritation. Creams and pessaries have only a local effect on the tissues of and around the vagina and vulva, and their use is associated with very low risk of heart disease or breast cancer. Blood levels of oestrogen rise slightly and women with a uterus should be given oral progesterone every three months to protect their uterine lining. Creams and pessaries do not improve bone density.

Combination oestrogen/progesterone

Oestrogen combined with a synthetic type of progesterone (progestogen) is the form of HRT recommended for women who have not had a hysterectomy. The preparations might be in the form of separate or combination tablets, or patches that have unvarying levels of oestrogen and progestogen. This is referred to as 'continuous' HRT. Alternatively, 'sequential' HRT contains oestrogen only in tablets or patches for about 14 days and then oestrogen with progestogen for another 10–14 days.

'Continuous'

Menopausal women are usually prescribed the 'continuous' type of HRT tablets or patches. With smaller and non-varying doses of progestogen, the endometrium tends to shrink, is less prone to cancerous change, and bleeding and 'periods' become a thing of the past. This type of HRT is used to treat menopausal symptoms or osteoporosis.

Some types of continuous HRT have been associated with an increased risk of harm. Research findings released in July 2002 from a study of conjugated oestrogens (from pregnant mare's urine) with medroxyprogesterone (a type of progestogen) revealed that risks outweighed benefits with this type regime. The trial was stopped after 5.2 instead of the planned 8.5 years.

The study showed an increasing risk of invasive breast cancer the longer this type of HRT was used, and that apparently healthy women developed more blood clots, strokes or heart attacks after a relatively short period of time. On the beneficial side, fracture risk was lower as was the risk of colon cancer.

Common combined tablets are Premia continuous, Menoprem continuous and Provelle 28. Individual tablets of Premarin can also be used with tablets of Provera.

Although the study identified one type of HRT as a problem, some doctors warn that all types of combination HRT might be risky and recommend short durations (6–12 months) to manage menopausal symptoms. They also warn against healthy women taking it to *prevent* heart disease or osteoporosis. Women with established osteoporosis should consider this type of HRT only after weighing up all risks and benefits—if risks in your case are high, other treatments for osteoporosis might be better (see page 45).

Other brand names of continuous HRT with different forms of oestrogen and progestogen are Kliovance and Kliogest tablets, and Estalis continuous patches.

'Sequential'
'Sequential' HRT refers to varying amounts of oestrogen and progestogens in tablets or patches. Tablets include Climen, Climen 28, Divina, Femoston, Menoprem, Premia 5 & 10, Trisequens and Trisequens forte; Estalis sequi and Estracombi are the patches. Sequential HRT will usually cause a 'period' and is usually given to peri-menopausal women short-term to treat menopausal symptoms.

Tablets are packaged like the Pill in blister packs with the first tablets containing oestrogen alone and the next containing oestrogen and progestogen. Sequential patches consist of oestrogen for two weeks then a combined patch for two weeks. Patches are changed every three to four days.

It is not clear whether sequential HRT (Menoprem, Premia 5 & 10; or Premarin for 28 days with Provera for

12–14 days) carries similar risks to the same type of continuous HRT. This is a less popular method of HRT—who wants a period at 60?—but some researchers are speculating that fewer days of progestogens may reduce risk and be safer for long-term use for those women with osteoporosis, for example. Remember though, there are risks with any long-term oestrogen use.

Testosterone

Testosterone creams or patches may soon be available for approved use. Testosterone is a 'male hormone' (androgen) that has been shown to help peri-menopausal and menopausal women with low sex drive and stamina, and altered moods.

Testosterone use can cause excess hair growth and acne, and so blood levels are checked to correct the dose and prevent this problem. Women should be cautious about embarking on this regime because some women with breast cancer have high blood levels of testosterone. It is unclear whether women using testosterone increase their chance of developing breast cancer and long-term studies are needed to establish risk.

'Bio-identical' HRT

Bio-identical HRT—chemically identical to hormones produced in your body—is a relative newcomer and has not undergone the sort of scrutiny other types of HRT have. It is available as gels, troches (held in the mouth) or capsules.

These hormones are made from precursors found in yams or soy plants and are said to have fewer side effects. However the many web pages extolling their virtues neatly side-step the issue of risks with long-term use. A woman's life-time exposure to oestrogens, natural or not, is known to be a risk factor in developing breast cancer, so be careful in your deliberations about taking these preparations, and be sure to understand the difference between no side effects and no risks.

Long-term studies will be needed to establish whether there are increased risks of developing breast and ovarian cancer, or heart and blood clotting. It is also uncertain whether bio-identical progesterone will adequately protect the uterine lining.

REASONS TO AVOID HRT

- Known or suspected pregnancy.
- Previous or active blood-clotting abnormality; heart disease, high blood pressure or stroke.
- Known or suspected breast cancer or oestrogen-dependent cancer.
- Undiagnosed, abnormal vaginal bleeding.
- Diabetes or epilepsy; diseases of the liver, kidney or pancreas. (You may experience a worsening of these conditions or additional side effects from HRT.)
- Recent or continuing cigarette smoking.

UNDESIRABLE EFFECTS OF HRT

Combined oestrogen and progestogen can cause **breast soreness**, **pain** and **swelling**. In rare cases, blood pressure might increase and so women should visit their doctor for a check up a few weeks after starting HRT and at least annually after that. Some conditions, such as fibroids and endometriosis, can worsen with oestrogen. If you have any of these, seek advice before starting HRT.

Migraines (caused by blood vessel spasm) that develop after starting HRT are a warning that you should stop. Some women, however, will experience total relief from migraines—it depends on your particular sensitivity.

Developing **gall bladder disease** is a possibility if you use HRT as tablets. When you take a tablet, the liver processes the hormones before they pass into the blood stream. This can concentrate the bile and cause stone formation in the gall bladder. Patches, gels and implants do not do this.

Bleeding between periods, after sex, or when not normally expected requires immediate investigation, whether you're on HRT or not. An ultrasound will usually be recommended to check the state of the endometrium. A hysteroscopy and biopsy of the endometrium may be needed to rule out endometrial cancer.

Other undesirable effects of HRT relate to cancer risk (see page 62), and the effect of hormones on the heart, blood vessels and blood clotting—see HRT and Your Heart, page 51.

GETTING OFF HRT

There are many reasons why you could decide to come off HRT. There may be no need to be on it any more, or you might be worried about developing breast cancer, or be diagnosed with a blood clot. Some women can come off HRT without any problems; others will get menopausal symptoms and need some help. Get some advice about coming off, or how to control symptoms. Here are some possible scenarios for coming off HRT:

Jennifer was taken off HRT after developing a blood clot following minor surgery. Her menopausal symptoms came flooding back: severe hot flushes, insomnia, she couldn't remember the right word for things, had memory loss and depressive moods. She started on dietary plant oestrogens as well as a herbal mixture containing *Cimicifuga racemosa*.

Initially, her symptoms were only partially controlled and she had a few difficult weeks during which she told her mother she was an interfering old bat who should be held in a high-security detention centre. After a few weeks of feeling miserable the herbal and dietary interventions kicked in, and Jennifer started to feel better. On the plus side, her mother still isn't speaking to her.

Wendy stopped taking HRT after five years and had no major problems except for a return of mild vaginal dryness. She used the cream containing *Cimicifuga racemosa* and evening primrose oil described on page 32, and apart from that Wendy has hardly noticed the difference.

OTHER OESTROGEN-LIKE DRUGS

Researchers are trying to find drugs to replace oestrogen with benefits on heart, blood, blood vessels, skin and brain, while avoiding negative consequences in the breast and uterus. Evista (raloxifene), a selective (o)estrogen receptor modulator (SERM), and Livial (tibolone), a synthetic steroid, are new drugs that aim to do just that.

Evista (raloxifene)

There are two different oestrogen receptors (the place where oestrogen and oestrogen-like substances dock before influencing the activity of a cell). Selective (o)estrogen receptor modulators (SERMs) are drugs that interact selectively with these receptors and elicit limited oestrogenic effects.

Evista is an SERM with oestrogen-like effects on bone. It is used for osteoporosis prevention, but is not as effective to *treat* osteoporosis as HRT or the bisphosphonates like Fosamax because it only reduces vertebral fractures, not hip fractures. Evista may worsen hot flushes, and won't help vaginal dryness, and so is not used for menopausal symptoms.

Evista blocks the effects of oestrogen in the breast and seems to protect against breast cancer, particularly in women with naturally high oestrogen levels. Research on the heart and blood vessels has been conflicting—it seems to increase the incidence of blood clots, but may reduce heart attacks and strokes in high-risk groups. Women with liver disease should not use Evista.

Tamoxifen (Genox, Nolvadex), the breast-cancer treatment and prevention drug, is also a SERM but has many side effects. It aggravates or causes hot flushes and vaginal dryness, and increases risk of blood clots and endometrial cancer. Its effect on bone is unclear.

Livial (tibolone)

Livial is a synthetic steroid that, once taken, is changed into hormone-like compounds that have varying effects from tissue to tissue—for example it acts like oestrogen to protect bone, relieve hot flushes and improve vaginal dryness; like progesterone to protect the endometrium; and like testosterone to increase sex drive.

Research has shown that, like tamoxifen, Livial does not stimulate breast cell growth. On the down side, it may increase cardiovascular problems. Trials are needed to study heart and blood clotting risks as well the incidence of breast or ovarian cancer to establish what constitutes safe long-term use of this drug.

CANCER, HRT AND OTHER OESTROGEN-LIKE DRUGS

Breast cancer

It is impossible to give precise figures on breast cancer risk because studies are designed and reported differently, using different types of HRT on women of different ages and with a variety of different risk factors. In fact, the breast cancer question is quite complex—as you might have guessed if you've seen a newspaper or TV lately. The issues are these:

- Breast cancer risk increases after five years or more on HRT, but some types of HRT carry more risk than others. Figures range from 20–40 per cent.
- Risk needs to be evaluated against an individual women's probability of developing breast cancer in the first place.
- An individual needs to assess her relative risk of breast cancer versus her risk of developing other complaints.

According to some studies, combined HRT (oestrogen with progestogen) may almost double the risk of breast cancer compared to oestrogen alone. HRT also makes breast tissue denser and so mammograms are harder to interpret—this is particularly so when a woman uses combined HRT. Evista and Livial seem to reduce breast cancer risk.

Breast cancer risk is increased by:
- obesity
- never having been pregnant and not having breast-fed (or pregnancy and breastfeeding later in life)
- taking the Pill as a teenager
- having a family history of breast cancer
- increased breast density on mammogram before starting HRT
- having diabetes

Women with any of these risks need to carefully consider their options before taking HRT.

However, women also need to look at what the 'relative' risk means for them if they need HRT for, say, osteoporosis. For example, one type of combined HRT was shown to increase risk of breast cancer by 26 per cent after five years. In real terms that means that each year 38 women out of 10 000 who take HRT will develop breast cancer compared to 30 women per 10 000 per year who do not. So some doctors will recommend that you consider HRT if your risk of breast cancer is low, but the risk of osteoporosis is high. Alternatively, you could look at the chapter on Healthy Bones after Menopause (page 37) for other dietary, lifestyle and drug suggestions.

Endometrial cancer

If you have not had a hysterectomy, any HRT preparation should include progestogens, or the risk of endometrial hyperplasia and endometrial cancer increases. The risk increases the longer you stay on the oestrogen-only regime, and remains higher for five or more years after stopping the treatment. Progestogens protect the uterine lining by causing it to shrink when used continuously, or to be shed when used sequentially. (See types of HRT page 53.)

Of the SERMs, tamoxifen, but not raloxifene (Evista) increases risk of endometrial cancer. Tibolone (Livial) seems to have a protective (progesterone-like) effect on the uterine lining.

Ovarian cancer

A woman's lifetime risk of developing ovarian cancer is 1.7 per cent. This means that, in a group of 100 women followed from birth to age 85, fewer than two would get ovarian cancer. (In comparison, about 13 women would get breast cancer.) However, according to a report released in July 2002 risk of ovarian cancer seems to increase amongst women who use oestrogen-only HRT by 80 per cent with 10 or more years of use, and by 220 per cent after 20 years. Translating this into lifetime risk, one to two more women per 100 on oestrogen-only HRT for 10 years or more, and about four more women per 100 taking this type of HRT for 20 years or more will get ovarian cancer.

Women taking sequential oestrogen and progestogens may also be at increased risk. Continuous, combined HRT appears to be safest. The effects of Evista and Livial on ovarian cancer risk are unknown because of a lack of long-term research.

Health Checklist for the Mid-life Woman

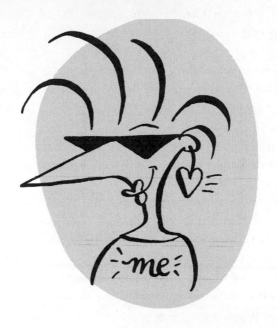

A monthly breast self-examination. Most doctors also recommend a mammogram every two years for women over 50.

A yearly check-up with your doctor including a pelvic exam, Pap test, breast exam, blood pressure check, and anything else you're worried about. These checks may need to be more frequent if there are problems.

Weight-bearing exercise for a minimum of 45 minutes at least every second day.

Calcium intake: 1500 milligrams a day. (Read the calcium info page in the Minerals section of the Self Care chapter.)

Magnesium intake: 800 milligrams a day. (Read the magnesium info page in the Minerals section of the Self Care chapter.)

Maintain your body weight at the middle to upper level of ideal weight range to protect your bones.

Book in for a bone density check if there's a strong family history of osteoporosis, or you have many risk factors. Re-check in two years.

A cholesterol check in your late forties or early fifties. Repeat as directed by your doctor if there's a family history of heart disease.

The Medical Approach

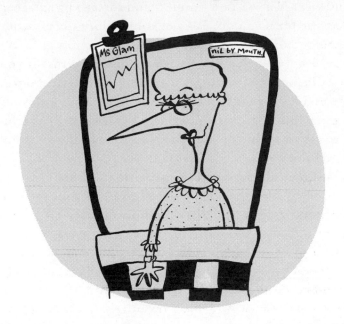

CHOOSING AND WORKING WITH YOUR DOCTOR

Doctors to avoid include ones who smoke during a consultation, ones who want to do nude hokey-pokey with you as part of the diagnostic process, doctors who say things like 'You leave it all up to me, dearie, you don't need to know the details', and doctors who insist that there is nothing valuable, under any circumstances, about natural therapies. Here are some ways to narrow the field:

- Find a sympathetic, smart, up-to-date general practitioner. Ask around, and then make up your own mind.
- Always ask if you don't understand something and keep asking until you do. It's not your failure to get it, it's the doctor's failure to make it clear for you.
- Take notes so you can review them afterwards. If you are being asked to absorb a lot of information at once, especially for the first time, you can walk out with your head in a fog, remembering afterwards only the bit where you think the doctor said, 'I'm afraid you've got myxomatosis'.
- First consultations with a specialist are usually half an hour, to allow the doctor to fully explore your medical history. Follow-up consultations will vary.
- Get a second opinion, or extra opinions, if you are unsure or unhappy with any recommendation by a general practitioner, specialist or surgeon.
- Always tell the doctor anything you think is relevant to your condition. This definitely includes other medications, herbs or supplements like vitamins you may be taking.
- Always follow the instructions on medicine exactly. Just because 10 milligrams makes you feel better, it doesn't mean 20 milligrams will be twice as good.
- When choosing a specialist for your particular problem, do as much research as you can about their experience, expertise and manner. Don't be afraid to try a few out before you decide.
- Find out if your surgeon is experienced in the latest specialised techniques, or is more of an all-round

gynaecologist. For complicated conditions, find a doctor who specialises in your problem.

- If you have surgery, the surgeon may visit you after the operation while you are still groggy. You may not remember the surgeon's report later. To be fully informed about what happened during your operation, and the implications for the future, get somebody to take notes for you then, organise a telephone call for a better time, or insist on an appointment as soon as you're up.

SCREENING

Any full check-up will involve a breast examination, a Pap test, a pelvic examination, and blood tests which are taken by the doctor or nurse and analysed in a pathology lab. Any vaginal bleeding after menopause must be investigated immediately by a doctor no matter how small, because it could be uterine cancer. Other causes of post-menopausal bleeding might be polyps or lesions on the cervix.

Here's what to expect and when to request a particular test:

Pelvic examination
When
Every year. (And yes, you still need pelvic exams if you're a lesbian or celibate.)

Why

Pain on movement of the organs, or other tell-tale signs such as an organ feeling 'fixed' when it's supposed to be more mobile can indicate endometriosis, infection or adhesions. It can also detect unusual swellings, enlargement of the ovaries, uterine fibroids, pregnancy, cysts and tumours. Ovarian cysts can happen at any age, but when they occur after the menopause it's best to have them surgically removed, as they are likely to be cancerous. Ovarian cysts cause few symptoms, if any, and are picked up by pelvic exam or ultrasound.

What

There are usually two stages to a pelvic 'exam'. Both are performed while you lie on your back on the couch in the doctor's office. It's okay to ask for a nurse to be there too. Here's the hard bit: with all that ferreting around going on down there you're supposed to relax. It's not exactly a calming experience, but it shouldn't hurt unless you tense up or there is something wrong. Sometimes the doctor will ask you to put your feet into 'stirrups'. (Try and resist the urge to say 'Giddy-up'.)

The doctor, wearing latex gloves over clean hands, will use a sterilised metal or plastic instrument called a speculum to very gently 'jack' open your vagina a little way so the doctor can look up the vagina and see the cervix. This is also a good time to have a Pap test, a case of 'While you're down there . . .'

For the full pelvic exam, the doctor will put two fingers inside the vagina so the tips of the fingers are in the area at the top of the vagina between the cervix and the wall of the vagina. The doctor's other hand will be placed on your lower abdomen. The doctor very gently wiggles fingertips to jostle some of your organs to feel if they are the right size and shape. The uterus and ovaries can be felt between the hands and, if you are relaxed (well, relatively relaxed), it is fairly easy to tell whether they are in the normal place, the right size and can move easily.

Now go and buy yourself a cup of tea and some chocolate cake.

Pap test
When
Once every two years regardless of your sexual preference, unless your doctor advises you to have one more often.

Why
A Papanicolaou smear test (named after the doctor who invented it) is used to screen for changes to the cells on the cervix, which may proceed to cervical cancer if untreated.

What
See the speculum procedure above in the pelvic exam section. (A new technique involves blowing air into the vagina instead but so far it hasn't really caught on.) After this, the doctor inserts a tiny, skinny wooden or plastic spatula to gently scrape cells from the surface of the cervix. The cells are then smeared onto a glass slide, given a squirt with hair spray (well, it looks like hair spray but they reckon it's a fixative) and sent to a pathology lab for

examination. (A new way of getting cells on the slide is being researched.) The procedure should be painless, but can be a little uncomfortable.

The cervical cells are examined under a microscope in a lab and graded according to the type of cells and whether they have undergone any changes. Pap tests can be inaccurate. When changes in cells are found in a Pap test, a colposcopy is often suggested. A colposcopy is a procedure in which a doctor looks up the vagina with a special telescope to see the cervix.

Pelvic ultrasound

When

Recommended by the doctor if you have bleeding between periods, unusually heavy periods or when a pelvic examination reveals a mass or that something is not quite right.

What

A type of imaging using high-frequency sound waves to show the inside of the pelvis. You will be lying down for the procedure.

Either the ultrasound operator will slide a little probe like a computer mouse around on the outside of your bare stomach, or if that won't get a good enough view, they will put a probe inside the vagina. The probe is usually shaped like a smooth pen with a small bulb shape on one end. It's not too big, and may be slightly uncomfortable when they move it around slightly, but it shouldn't hurt.

The image is projected on a small screen. The ultrasound operator will be able to explain to you what is being seen—otherwise, you're thinking the TV's gone on the blink or something and they're going, 'Ye Gads! It's an ovarian follicle!'

Breast checks
When
Every month after each period by you and an annual check by a doctor. Most women detect breast changes themselves. They know the 'normal' feel of their own breasts and are in an unique position to detect change and detect it early.

Why
You're looking for lumps or any changes in breast tissue. About 80 per cent of breast lumps are not cancerous, but even when a breast lump is caused by cancer, the earlier it is found, the better the outlook.

What
Breast examination involves two phases: visual and physical examination of the breast tissue. Do it after every period, and after menopause, once a month. You need to get to know intimately the feel of your breasts and report ANY changes to a doctor. Now we could print a very involved chart here, but really, we'd prefer you went to the doctor and got a lesson in how to do it properly, because it's easy once you know how. To jog your memory, pick up a pamphlet while you're there or get one from the Women's Health Care Centre in your area (contact details are at the back of the book).

Mammogram

When

These are recommended every two years for women 50 and over, and more often for women who have had breast cancer or a strong possibility of developing breast cancer (for example a genetic predisposition).

What

The mammogram operator will place one of your breasts on a metal plate and then bring another plate down on the top of your breast, squashing it as far as it can. A 'photograph' is then taken of the breast tissue, and that image will help a specialist identify areas of concern, including lumps that must be investigated. A mammogram will not be able to identify whether a lump is benign or malignant but can give the doctor a fairly clear idea of what type of lump has been discovered.

Ultrasound of breast

When

Performed in addition to a mammogram to determine the size and location of cysts or breast lumps.

What

This is a type of imaging using high-frequency sound waves to look at soft tissue structures in the breast such as cysts or lumps. A sticky gel is smoothed over the breast and a small instrument, something similar to a computer mouse, is moved over the breast. It doesn't hurt and is frequently used to tell whether a lump detected with a mammogram is a breast cancer or cyst. For a definite diagnosis, either a needle biopsy (aspiration of cells or fluid from the lump) or a lumpectomy will need to be performed.

Natural Therapies

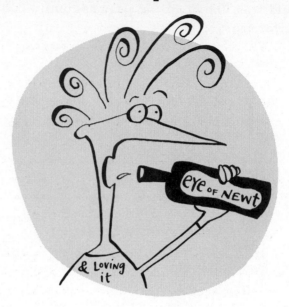

eye OF NEWt

& loving it

CHOOSING AND WORKING WITH YOUR NATURAL THERAPIST

Natural therapists to avoid are ones who have to work sitting under a pyramid for the 'vibes'; ones who insist that they are 'healers' (Blue heelers, maybe); ones who explain that most of their knowledge is based on 'intu-itive' messages from the Great Beyond; and ones who say there is no value, under any circumstances, in scientific medicine. Here are some hints on how to narrow the field:

- Familiarise yourself with the different disciplines of natural therapy, and decide which kind of practitioner might suit you best.
- Find out what professional qualifications the therapist has, how recent their training is and how they keep abreast, and what professional organisations your therapist belongs to.
- Many natural therapists prescribe herbs. It is best if herbs are prescribed by a full member of the National Herbalists' Association of Australia.
- Your practitioner should, at least, be affiliated with the major governing group for their discipline. (The National Herbalists' Association of Australia requires 700 hours of relevant study for membership; equivalent State bodies also require 700 hours, the Australian Natural Therapists' Association requires 700 hours study in an approved course; and the Australian Traditional Medicine Society requires a specific number of hours for each discipline.)
- Regardless of their qualifications, you have to like and trust your therapist. Don't be afraid to shop around.
- Try to find a natural therapist who specialises in your problem.
- Any treatment must target the underlying cause, not just the symptoms: you need a full diagnosis as well as treatment. For example, if you have heavy bleeding, don't accept a preparation to stop it without knowing the gynaecological cause. If you simply mask important symptoms, you might be hiding an underlying problem that your body is trying to warn you about.

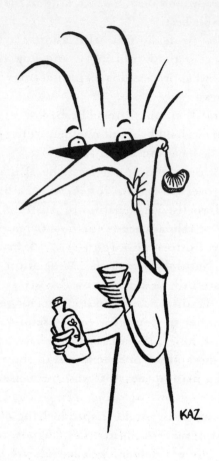

Some herbal concoctions taste weird

This means you may have to have medical tests then return to the natural therapist armed with the results.

- Some crucial examinations are not performed by natural therapists and referral to a doctor is needed. The results of the tests can be used by a natural therapist, or a doctor, or both, as a base for their diagnosis and treatment. These include routine screens like Pap tests and breast exams; gynaecological examinations which are performed vaginally and involve internal 'examination' of the pelvic organs; pathology tests such as blood tests, swabs or urine tests; radiological examinations such as ultrasounds and X-rays; and diagnostic operations such as a laparoscopy, a procedure used to look around the pelvic organs, usually searching for problems like blocked Fallopian tubes, endometriosis or cysts of some kind.
- Be suspicious of practitioners who prescribe vast amounts of herbs or supplements from their clinic at inflated prices. Four different preparations is a fairly average prescription. If you go home with a plastic bag with 15 different pills, powders and potions, a bunch of pussy willows and seven sacks of dandelion tea, you should be asking why you need it all. It is quite proper for a natural therapist to dispense from their own clinic, just make sure that if they sell you over-the-counter products, for example, Blackmore's, that their price is competitive with say, your local supermarket. This goes for health food shops too.
- Be wary of any doctor or natural therapist who has a hard and fast pet theory which they apply to all situations—examples of these are people who claim that

most disorders, from period pain to exhaustion are caused only by the liver, or stress, or dehydration, or toxicity, or the fact that the moon in June was in Pisces.

- Always tell the natural therapist anything you think is relevant to your condition. This definitely includes other medications you're on, including drugs, herbs or supplements (including vitamins).
- Always follow the instructions on herbal prescriptions and supplements exactly. Never assume that just because something is 'natural' you can take as much as you want to, or vary the recommended doses. Like drugs, under some circumstances, herbs can be dangerous.
- If you are not happy with the results of treatment, seek a second or further opinion.
- Don't expect a natural therapist to be able to 'cure' everything. There are some conditions which are not satisfactorily treated by natural methods.

Self Care

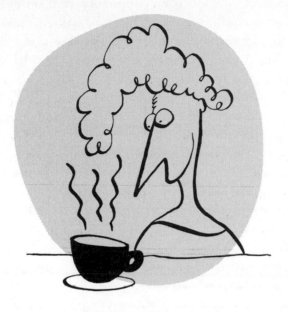

Caring for yourself is not about self-diagnosis or treatment without proper guidance. It does involve learning to recognise signs and symptoms to prevent illness. If you learn more about your body it will help you to recognise early signs of any change that may need attention. Here are some important things to remember about looking after yourself:

- Get tested. See the mid-life woman's checklist on page 65.
- Learn to 'listen' to your body. This doesn't mean a hippy-drippy psychic version of the stethoscope, it

means if you really feel like there's something wrong, there probably is. Don't ignore warning signs and symptoms. And get another opinion if you're not happy with your doctor's comments or examination.

- Take prescriptions from doctors and natural therapists exactly as recommended, and make sure that each of your health care providers knows what the other ones are doing.

- Don't self-diagnose, don't prescribe yourself drugs or herbs, and don't wear your underpants on your head. You'll look stupid.

- Be as well informed as possible about any condition or disease you are dealing with. Don't just read one book, or one theory, or listen to one piece of advice. It can be tempting to fasten onto one reason or theory to explain everything, because it's simple.

- Be willing to accept that self care can only go so far with some conditions, and further or more complex treatment may be necessary.

- Remember that even if you are doing all the right things with your diet and lifestyle, you may still need to manage an illness in other ways. Don't be mad at yourself, just think how much worse it would be if you had a packet of Peter Stuyvesants and a Coke for breakfast every day.

FOOD FOR HEALTH

About the closest most doctors get to asking about your diet is to say 'Are you eating well?' To which you can reply, 'Oooh yes, doctor', meaning that you skip breakfast, have eight Tim Tams for lunch and usually eat the weight of a small hatchback each evening, mostly from the food groups entitled 'lard' and 'utter crap'.

Natural therapists are more likely to pry into your eating habits and suggest some specific changes. Let's be frank: eating properly doesn't mean you'll never get sick, but it will make you healthier and less likely to get sick. And it means you recover more quickly. Not that we're the type to say 'Oh, you've just had your leg amputated. Half a cup of dandelion tea a day and that'll grow right back in no time.'

There are also some specific foods and combinations of foods which can help with recognised conditions. So we've included a couple of therapeutic short-term diets. These are not like the short-term weight-loss diets and should be used under the supervision of your health practitioner.

Here's a 'top 20' of sensible suggestions for healthy eating. It's a general guide which you can use to introduce healthy changes to the way you eat. Don't try to change everything at once, don't regard the hints as a set of hard and fast rules and don't start faffing around the place weighing bits of food and stressing about whether you need another 76.4 grams of tofu before Thursday, or you'll bore yourself to death.

20 DIET HINTS

1. Eat varied and interesting food
We're not talking about sitting down to a bowl of chaff three times a day with half a mung bean for morning tea.

83

Don't eat foods you hate just because 'they're good for you'. Lots of different kinds of food is the go. And relax. You're not going to explode if you have a chocolate bickie every now and then.

2. Drink plenty of fluids every day

Otherwise you'll shrivel up like a dried apricot and blow away. Well, not quite. But you need at least 2 litres of water a day, and more when it's hot or you're exercising. By the time you have a dry mouth, dehydration has already started, so don't wait until you're really thirsty. Fluids should be varied and should not come only from coffee, tea and fluffy duck cocktails. Two or three glasses of plain water, preferably filtered, throughout the day are essential. Fruit juices should be diluted because of their high sugar content.

3. Eat fresh and organic foods

Fresh is best—there are fewer preservatives, the food is less likely to be rancid, nutrient levels are higher and it tastes better. It's easier to see if fresh food has been spoiled or is old and past its 'use by' date. The closer you can get to the original source of the food, the better. This doesn't mean you have to go out and pick everything yourself, it means make sure your best pal is not the can-opener. Where possible, buy organic foods to minimise exposure to chemicals.

4. 'Therapeutic' diets are temporary

A therapeutic diet is prescribed with a particular goal—say, lowering cholesterol, improving anaemia, getting rid of thrush, or calming an irritable bowel. Therapeutic diets should only be used until the result is achieved, and always under the supervision of a health practitioner. Many of them don't contain the required nutrients, kilojoules or balance for extended use. If you react badly, go off it: therapeutic diets are not appropriate for all conditions or people.

5. Eat 5 to 7 different vegies and 3 fruits a day

Vegies and fruit contain a good range of vitamins, minerals, trace elements, essential fatty acids, anti-oxidants and fibre. Women in the forties and over need fibre and anti-oxidants to reduce risk of cancer and heart disease. Particular foods can also help to target particular problems. Cabbages and tomatoes reduce cancer risk; legumes contain plant oestrogens; bitter components flush the gall bladder; fruit pectin lowers cholesterol; and celery lowers blood pressure and reduces acid build-up in joints.

The old habit of 'a huge hunk of meat and three vegies boiled to death' should be abandoned with a sense of wild glee. To retain the most nutrients, it's best to cook vegies by steaming, stir-frying or baking. Every day you should eat from two to three different orange, red or yellow vegetables, a minimum of two green vegetables, at least one of the cabbage family such as broccoli or cabbage, and some garlic or onion for their cancer-preventing and blood vessel protecting properties.

Fruit should be limited to three pieces a day because it doesn't seem to have the same energy-improving qualities of vegies (this may be because fruits are generally lower in minerals and higher in sugars). Fruit should preferably be eaten whole and not juiced, because juicing reduces the fibre content.

6. Main energy foods should be complex carbohydrates

Carbohydrates are energy foods. When eaten as whole foods (such as brown instead of white rice) they are known as complex carbohydrates. Less useful refined carbohydrate comes from foods like white bread. The main part of the diet should be based on complex carbohydrates from whole grains and legumes, dried beans and peas, nuts and seeds, soya products and some of the root vegies like potato, carrots and sweet potato. Common good energy foods include breakfast cereals and muesli, bread, rice, beans, tofu, pasta and potato. They can lower blood cholesterol, stabilise blood sugar, regulate the bowel, reduce the appetite and ensure a good supply of regular energy. The slow energy release leads to greater stamina and fewer energy slumps. They are important for menopausal women because they are high in fibre and many also contain plant oestrogens.

Carbo combos
Complex carbohydrates contain plenty of fibre and some of the amino acids which make up proteins. They can be combined in a meal so that they become a substitute for

animal protein. Carbohydrate-combining should be used by vegetarians to make sure that they get enough protein every day. The common combinations are:

- grains with beans: tofu and rice (Asia), lentils and rice (India), tortilla and beans (Mexico)
- grains and nuts: peanuts and rice (Southern Asia), nut butters and bread (bread-eating countries), rice and cashews (Asia)
- beans and seeds: sesame seed paste and beans (Middle East).

Many people instinctively cook like this or follow traditional recipes which incorporate food combinations. Combining carbohydrates gives all of the energy benefits of protein, as well as the positive benefits of complex carbohydrates without a high animal fat intake.

7. Eat enough fibre

Fibre should be included in the diet to aid with lowering of blood fats (cholesterol) and oestrogens; to reduce the incidence of gall bladder disease and colon cancer; for weight loss; and to treat constipation. Fibre is specifically important for women because it reduces the risk of oestrogen-dependent cancers, including breast cancer as well as bowel cancer.

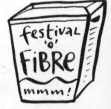

The best source of dietary fibre is from whole foods, but occasionally it may be necessary to use processed fibre products (like wheat bran, oat or rice bran), to effectively treat some diseases. Wheat bran, 'fibrous' vegetables (like celery and carrot), potato and other root vegies, tofu, legumes and linseed meal are all good sources of fibre.

The recommended daily intake for fibre is 30 grams for an adult from whole foods, and not as fibre-only breakfast cereals. This could be achieved by eating the following in the one day: five serves of whole-grain or legume products (such as two slices of bread, a cup of cooked beans, a cup of brown rice, and a cup of break-fast cereal) and five serves of different vegetables and three pieces of fruit.

8. Eat fewer 'bad fats' and more 'good fats'

Fat is the devil! It causes heart disease! It turns you into a hideous gargoyle! You'll get cholesterol problems and your head will fall off! And now they've invented a synthetic oil with no absorbable fat which causes 'anal leakage'. So what! It hasn't got any fat! Hmmm. It's just an inkling, but maybe it's time to get a bit less hysterical.

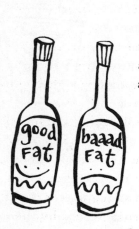

The fact is that if you cut out ALL fats you'll have more problems than when you started. There's good ones and bad ones. We all need a reason-able level of fats in our diet. They are essential for the production of sex and adrenal hormones, for the health of our skin and mucous membranes. When the right fats are eaten, they protect against high cholesterol and heart disease, skin and period problems, and a whole lot else.

Bad fats

- An overall reduction of all fats is good.
- Cut down on saturated fats—they're in animal products (pork, beef, lamb and dairy products) and in the tropical oils (coconut and palm oils). Excessive saturated fat intake is linked to heart disease, obesity and an increased risk of some cancers.
- Cut down on the Omega-6 polyunsaturated fats. High levels of Omega-6 polyunsaturated fats are found in cooking oils and margarine.
- Avoid trans-fatty acids. These are in oils which are processed to become solid, like margarine and vegetable shortening. The high temperature process changes the oil molecule, and destroys essential fatty acids ('good fats'). Trans-fatty acids interfere with the production of the useful group of prostaglandins which prevent PMS, period pain and a heap of inflammatory problems.
- Look for 'contains hydrogenated fats' on labels and avoid it.
- Overall, too many fats, sugars, alcohol or carbohydrates are converted into triglycerides which increase the risk of heart disease, kidney failure, high blood pressure and cancer.
- To reduce risk of heart disease, cholesterol-containing foods should be minimised, but the 'good fats' must be increased as well, to have the right effect. Cholesterol is used by the body to make hormones and other bits and pieces, so you shouldn't cut it out altogether. It is found in all animal fats but not vegetable fats. (The body makes its own cholesterol,

partly from eaten cholesterol, and partly as a response to eating other saturated fats.)

Good fats
To let the good fats do their work properly, you need to cut down on the bad fats, which can interfere with their work.

- Mono-unsaturated fats are the good vegetable oils to cook with and are more stable than polyunsaturated fats when they are exposed to heat, light or oxygen. Olive oil is the best-known mono-unsaturated oil and when used as a substitute for saturated fats, helps to lower cholesterol and reduce the risk of heart disease.
- Fatty acids are necessary for the normal function and development of most tissues including the kidney, liver, blood vessels, heart and brain. A deficiency leads to excessive scaliness of the skin, reduced growth rates and infertility in both males and females; and can also cause a greater susceptibility to infections, fragile red blood cells and difficulty in making prostaglandins.

Omega-3 fatty acids
The Omega-3 fatty acids are particular polyunsaturated fats. Suffice to say that we all need Omega-3 fatty acids, which are known as EPA (eicosapentaenoic acid), DHA (docosahexaenoic acid). ALA (alpha linolenic acid) is an essential fatty acid which the body cannot make itself from other fatty acids.

To keep your prostaglandins in balance, and to control imbalance-related conditions, like blood fat abnormalities, wound healing and to improve mood—all sorts of things—you need to regularly eat foods rich in Omega-3 fatty acids.

To make the right prostaglandins, you need to include these Omega-3s in your diet:

Linseeds or linseed (flax seed) oil. These are very rich sources of ALA. You can take 1 to 2 tablespoons of ground linseeds a day. To help digestion and absorption, linseeds should be ground in a coffee grinder used only for seeds, never coffee (or mortar and pestle if you're feeling rustic), and can be sprinkled on muesli or tossed in a smoothie. They must be refrigerated in airtight containers or scoffed immediately after grinding. (Don't bother buying the pre-ground linseeds in packets at health food shops.) Alternatively, you could take 2 teaspoons of linseed/flax seed oil a day to be stored the same way. When served as recommended, linseed oil has 60 per cent ALA.

Pumpkin seeds (15 per cent ALA); **canola oil** (10 per cent); **mustard seed oil** (10 per cent); **soya bean oil** (7 to 9 per cent). Walnut oil also has moderate levels; and dark green leafy vegetables have small amounts. These fatty acids tend to go off and must be refrigerated in opaque bottles. No ALA oils should be cooked.

Oily fish. The best fish to eat are cold-water and oilier fish. Menopausal women should include some of these fish in at least four meals a week. 'Oily' fish are often deep sea fish, where they've needed a bit of protection from the cold.

If you can't buy fresh fish, get it in cans, although the benefits will be less obvious. Choose from: gemfish, blue mackerel, sea mullet, blue warehou, silver warehou, yellowtail kingfish, King George whiting, redfish, tuna, sardines, herring, pilchards, Atlantic salmon, silver trevally, luderick, ocean trout, blue eye, golden perch, blue grenadier, and rainbow trout.

Fish oil supplements are usually capsules which include 18 per cent EPA and 12 per cent DHA and are made from fish oils or fish liver oils. Cod liver and halibut liver oils, however, also contain vitamins A and D, which means that they are no good for the long term at large doses. (It's dangerous to take vitamin A supplements if you're pregnant.) Fish oils have a long list of therapeutic effects which includes reducing heart disease; reducing arthritic inflammation; and an improvement in allergy-related conditions such as asthma and eczema.

Omega-6 fatty acids
Linoleic acid. Eat some of this when you can. It helps with dryness of skin and eyes which is common after menopause, as well as improving symptoms related to hormone imbalance in the peri-menopause. Linoleic acid is found in seed and vegetable oils, as well as most nuts, and organ meats. Coconut oil and dairy products contain very low levels of linoleic acid. Although the levels are low compared to seeds, any dark green vegetable is a source of linoleic acid. Linoleic acid is an essential fatty acid. Essential, in this case, merely means that you must eat them because the body won't manufacture them by itself.

There's lots of linoleic acid in seed oils: safflower oil (75 per cent); sunflower oil (60 to 70 per cent); walnut oil (60 per cent); corn oil (55 per cent); soya bean oil (50 per cent); peanut oil (35 per cent) and olive oil (8 per cent).

Evening primrose oil, blackcurrant seed oil and borage seed oil are also rich sources of linoleic acid.

Gamma-linolenic acid. Gamma-linolenic acid (GLA) is the building block from which the body makes the prostaglandins that reduce inflammation, stop pain and activate the immune system. GLA is found in the oils of evening primrose, blackcurrant, safflower, sunflower, hemp, soybean, pumpkin seed, borage seed and walnut. These seed oils have been shown to reduce sore breasts and the severity of other PMS symptoms.

Evening primrose, star flower oil and blackcurrant seed oil are available as capsules which contain beneficial amounts of GLAs as well as linolenic acid.

Cooking and storing hints for oils

- Mono-unsaturated fats are the best oils for cooking. Pour them into a pan that's already hot to reduce heating time. Never re-use oils.
- Don't cook in other oils. Heating induces irreversible changes to many oils which leads to oxidation or free radical formation. Foods can be cooked in just a little water, or even 'dry fried' in a non-stick pan. Fish, eggs and vegetables can be poached in water, or a fruit or vegetable puree, and fish and vegetables can be baked rather than roasted in oil.

- Add oils to food after cooking as salad dressings or sauces.
- Eat more cold-pressed oils of linseed, safflower and canola as tablespoon doses once or twice a day or added to a seed breakfast or muesli used in salad dressings, poured onto cooked food or mixed with yoghurt in a ratio of about one part oil to five parts yoghurt.
- Make your own spreads with avocado, tahini, yoghurt, chickpeas, nut butters or vegetable-based dips instead of margarine or butter.
- Buy oils manufactured without damage to the goodies ('cold-pressed', 'unrefined' or 'mechanically extracted') and in opaque glass bottles. All oils and oil-containing foods should be refrigerated. Otherwise they have a habit of going off.

9. Eat dairy products in moderation

Many people are sensitive to dairy products, or at least some aspects of them, and some natural therapists recommend that they not be eaten at all, while dietitians see the enormous potential for nutrients, especially calcium, and recommend a high intake. What's going on? Are they good for us or what? Well, they're okay, if you eat the

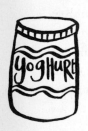

low-fat varieties, unless you have a dairy intolerance, and even then, it is likely you can eat yoghurt. Menopausal women need several serves of dairy per day, preferably low fat and high calcium. White cheeses, parmesan and yoghurt are the best sources and seem to be better tolerated than creamier, fattier cheeses.

Yoghurt is an important food. It is easily digestible, provides good bacteria which makes the gut work properly, has more calcium than milk, and may help to reduce the risk of breast and other oestrogen-dependent cancers. It is also well tolerated by those with a dairy or lactose intolerance. Read the label to make sure a yoghurt has live cultures; many of the snack-type yoghurts don't, especially the flavoured and 'fruit yoghurts'. Get low-fat, no-sugar brands.

Don't forget bones need magnesium too, if calcium is to be properly retained, and dairy foods don't have much magnesium.

10. Eat plant oestrogens

Plant oestrogens, which are explained fully towards the end of this section, are structurally similar to animal oestrogen and are found in a large number of common foods and medicinal plants. Eating plant oestrogens is associated with a reduced incidence of oestrogen-related disease such as endometriosis, and breast and endometrial cancer. Plant oestrogens also lower blood cholesterol and blood pressure.

11. Eat enough protein regularly

When people go on 'healthy' or 'weight-loss' diets, they often drastically reduce or stop most of their protein intake. Protein is found in animal products such as meat, eggs, fish, milk and cheese, and also in the vegetable proteins such as tofu. Neither type is better or worse, unless you're a vegetarian.

Vegetarians (lacto-ovo), for example, can obtain protein from eating vegetable proteins, dairy products and eggs; vegans get it from eating combinations of vegetables. It's harder to get iron and zinc, and for the vegan, to get vitamin B12 as well. The advantage of being a vegetarian is a lower intake of fat and less likelihood of developing many of the chronic degenerative diseases; the disadvantage is a tendency to anaemia and fatigue.

Meat-eaters have an advantage when it comes to iron and zinc intake. Iron in meat is easier to absorb and it is present in much greater quantities. Many women in Australia eat far less than the recommended daily intake for zinc. Animal protein is also of a better quality and meat-eaters can have a more relaxed attitude to nutrient intake and still maintain energy levels. On the down side, eating meat increases the intake of saturated fats and the risk of a number of diseases, such as heart disease and cancer. Deep-sea fish is better because it contains high levels of essential fatty acids as well as protein. This means you have to ask the fishmonger if the fish is from the deep sea. (Or there's the list of oily fish in the previous Good Fats section.)

For those who do eat meat, protein can come from (preferably chemical-free) lean, red meat in small quantities, some organic chicken without the skin, plenty of fish, no more than three eggs a week and low-fat dairy products. At least some of the protein should come from properly combined vegetable sources. How to combine them is explained in point six on carbohydrates.

You should eat about 45–55 grams of protein each day. Here are some levels of protein in food:

100 grams of meat	20–25 grams
100 grams of seafood	15–20 grams
1 cup beans/legumes	7.5–15 grams
1 cup whole grains	5–12 grams
1 cup milk or yoghurt	8 grams
1 egg	6 grams
30 grams of cheese	6–8 grams
1 cup vegies or fruit	2–4 grams

12. Know your minerals

The key ones for women are in the next section, astonishingly enough entitled 'Minerals'.

13. Eat foods in season

Apart from the ludicrous price of foods that are out of season or imported (Darling, how marvellous! These July raspberries are only $6000 a punnet!) there's another reason to buy what's locally available at the right time of year.

All fruits and vegetables can be assigned with certain qualities in the same way that medicinal herbs are. Summer foods are generally juicy and light, winter foods tend to be dense and compact with lots of carbohydrate and protein. In summer, moist, easily digested raw foods make sense, but in winter they don't provide enough carbohydrate to counterbalance the energy expenditure needed to stay warm.

Winter foods should be mainly beans, legumes and root vegetables; salads can be made from root vegetables and cabbage. These are warming and comforting foods on a cold winter's day.

Most summer fruits and vegetables have cooling

properties—melons are particularly cooling, while bananas, which tend to be dense and compact, are warming. Eat stuff that seems instinctively right for that time of the year.

14. Vary the flavours

There are five main flavours in the diet: bitter, sweet, sour, salty and spicy or pungent. Australians traditionally rely heavily on the sweet and salty flavours, but other cultures include all or most of the flavours in their cooking as a matter of course—Thai food, for example, is cooked with the addition of salty, sweet, spicy and sour flavours. Each of the flavours has subtle effects on digestion and health.

Bitter

As we get older digestive function and gastric acid production tends to deteriorate, leading to, among other things, poor mineral uptake. Bitter foods improve digestion and bowel function by stimulating the bile flow. Bitter green vegetables and radicchio, chicory, dandelion leaves and silverbeet are often included in the European diet to aid digestion. (Spinach is not a 'bitter' because it doesn't taste bitter.) Grapefruit is sour and bitter, and the old practice of having half a grapefruit before a fatty breakfast such as bacon and eggs makes a lot of sense. (Almost as much as not eating the fatty breakfast every morning.) Dandelion coffee is a gentle and effective mild bitter that is available as a beverage. It is available as a beverage that tastes (like bat wee, if you asked one of the authors of this book, but we shall draw a tactful veil over this fact) good mixed with soya milk.

Spicy

Warming spices in the diet improve sluggish digestion and are particularly useful for complaints of the upper gastro-intestinal tract such as nausea, burping and indigestion. Ginger, cardamom, cumin and coriander are all useful—ginger tea is particularly helpful for nausea. (Cut two or three bits of fresh knobbly ginger root, about 2 centimetres long, throw them in a teapot, add boiling water and let it steep for a couple of minutes.) These spices can be brewed in ordinary black tea to assist with digestion. Warming spices are useful for those who feel cold, have difficulties with cold weather, or catch colds easily.

Sour

Sour foods are drying and can be used to stop snuffy noses. For some people, sweet foods cause phlegm or catarrh and sour foods can reverse the process. Many sour foods, such as citrus fruit, are useful to protect the mucous membranes from infections. Sour foods also aid digestion.

15. Don't stuff yourself silly

Overeating (to be perfectly obvious) is linked to obesity and a shorter life expectancy. The digestive tract is chronically overburdened and the incidence of gall bladder disease increases. The heart has to work harder and the risk of high blood pressure also increases.

16. Don't argue with your food

Eat foods which agree with you. Listen to your body and act accordingly. Some common diets cause obvious problems in some people, such as abdominal upsets, diarrhoea, or fatigue. And sometimes your body decides it used to like something but now it's gone right off it.

Raw food diets can be a problem, for example, because raw food is quite difficult to digest. Bloating, wind or even diarrhoea can lead to a depletion of nutrients and ill health. Trading one health problem (for example, shocking wind) for another (like being overweight) doesn't make sense.

17. Limit sugar and salt

Sugar

All types of sugar should be minimised, including brown and unrefined sugars; as well as the foods which are prepared with sugar and processed food with added sugar (this includes stuff like tinned beans, even).

Salt

Salt intake is associated with high blood pressure and increases the excretion of minerals in the urine. Most sodium (salt) enters the diet in manufactured foods, not through adding salt during cooking or at the table. Salt should be limited to around 3–5 grams daily. A high salt intake increases the risk of osteoporosis.

18. Limit caffeine

Caffeine-containing drinks contain highly active substances known as xanthines. (Xanthines, while sounding like a girlfriend of Xena, Warrior Princess, are actually alkaloids which have diverse effects in the body.) Caffeine is in coffee, tea, cocoa and chocolate.

Caffeine increases anxiety, aggravates insomnia, helps to waste minerals and increases blood pressure. Excessive caffeine intake is also linked with a number of common gynaecological conditions including endometriosis, fibroids, PMS and benign breast disease—all from the equivalent of two cups of coffee every day. 'Plunger' coffee has the least harmful effects. Boiled coffee should be completely avoided if there are problems with high cholesterol levels.

19. Cut down on alcohol

Women are more affected by alcohol for longer periods of time than men. Women have a lower body water content and so alcohol is less diluted. They also metabolise (break down) alcohol more slowly because they have a smaller liver cell mass than men. This is why there are different government health warnings for women and men.

Two standard alcoholic drinks in less than an hour will take a woman to the legal blood alcohol limit for driving, but this figure may be influenced by hormonal fluctuations of the menstrual cycle (around the period and ovulation, alcohol is thought to be metabolised more slowly), by cigarette smoking and by diet.

Excess alcohol consumption has been linked to cancers, hypertension, heart disease, foetal abnormalities, and liver disease. A host of other more subtle health problems are caused or aggravated by alcohol. Some are caused by depletion of minerals such as calcium, magnesium, potassium and zinc, and vitamins A, C and the B complex, especially B1. The National Health and Medical Research Council have made the following recommendations for women:

- Women should limit drinking to two standard drinks or 20 grams of absolute alcohol per day and have two or three alcohol-free days a week to give the liver some recovery time.
- More than two drinks a day or 14 drinks a week is officially considered dangerous. Any more than that and you're officially damaging yourself.
- Don't drink at all if you're pregnant. Also, if you do get legless drunk, don't go for the 'hair of the dog' and start all over again. Give your body free time to get over it: about two days between drinks is recommended.

20. Eat more serenely

A common cause of digestive problems and poor nutrient uptake, is the practice of eating in the car, watching TV or on the run. Meal times need to be a little sacred; a time set aside to think about food, be with family, friends or self. Taking time to chew food thoroughly is an essential beginning to good digestion. Avoid unnecessary argument or conflict and try not to eat when upset or in pain. If possible wait until you feel better. Most importantly, enjoy what you are eating. If you happen to eat some junk food, enjoy it, then get on with wholesome eating.

WHAT TO AIM TO EAT EVERY DAY

Vegies
A minimum of five to seven different vegetables daily; from at least two green and two orange, yellow or red vegetables. Darker vegies are better for trace minerals and anti-oxidants.

Fruit
Choose pieces from three different fresh, seasonal fruits.

Complex carbohydrates or whole grains and beans/legumes
Include four to five serves of grains such as wheat, rice, corn, hulled millet and/or beans such as chickpeas, lentils, red kidney beans, lima beans, soya beans and soya products. A serve is equivalent to a slice of bread, one cup of cooked grain or beans, or one medium-sized to large potato.

Yoghurt and cultured milks
Include at least one cup of low-fat yoghurt daily. If sensitive to cow's milk, include soya, goat's or sheep's yoghurt instead. Yoghurts should contain live cultures.

Fibre

Fibre should come from whole foods such as grains, nuts, seeds, fruit and vegetables and not from fibre-only bran-based, commercial breakfast cereals.

Fats and oils

Include three teaspoons of raw seed oils in the diet daily, such as flax, canola, safflower or sunflower, but try to avoid margarine. To make 'better butter' mix equal quantities by weight of a good quality olive oil and butter. Keep refrigerated.

Seeds and nuts

Seeds: linseeds, sesame seeds, sunflower seeds, pumpkin seeds.

Nuts: almonds, hazelnuts, walnuts, pecans, cashews, pine nuts and peanuts.

Nuts and seeds have a high ratio of oils and should be kept to a maximum of half a cup a day. For an equivalent amount of fibre and protein substitute with one of the grain or bean servings, as well as one of the teaspoons of oil.

Protein

Protein is found in meat, fish, eggs, dairy products and properly combined vegetable proteins. Some protein should be taken with every meal.

Calcium-containing foods

Menopausal women need 1500 milligrams daily so be sure to add some dairy, especially yoghurt, and try sardines, tofu, and green leafies. Look on the check list on page 117 for more sources.

MEAL SUGGESTIONS

Morning kick-start

Start the day with one of these:
- the juice of a lemon diluted in a glass of warm water
- half a grapefruit
- citrus juice
- a whole piece of fruit.

(We're not suggesting that's your whole breakfast, but have one of them before anything else. It will wake up your digestive process.)

Breakfast ideas
- Home-made muesli: raw oatmeal, rice flakes, puffed millet, sunflower seeds, linseeds, sultanas, chopped almonds or cashews, dried paw paw, coconut and chopped pumpkin seeds. Add low-fat cow's milk, yoghurt or soya milk, and chopped fresh fruit.
- Fresh fruit in season with yoghurt and seeds or chopped nuts.
- Wholegrain bread, toasted with nut butter, hommos, low-fat cheese, miso, alfalfa or other sprouts. You don't need butter with these spreads. Avoid honey and jams.

- Cooked cereal such as oatmeal, millet meal, brown rice or buckwheat, with added seeds or soya grits. Add milk of choice and fruit or a bit of honey.
- Energy drink: blend together low-fat yoghurt with either fresh fruit of your choice or fruit juice (about half and half), and add a teaspoon each of rice bran, ground linseeds, almond meal, wheatgerm, and sunflower seeds.

Lunch ideas

- Wholegrain bread sandwich with a mixture of salad vegies. Include a bit of protein such as tuna, salmon, sardines, egg, low-fat cheese, or hommos. Marinated tofu is also good in a sandwich.
- Salad of mixed vegies such as lettuce salad, coleslaw, tabouli salad, grated beetroot, tomatoes, carrot or celery. Protein should be included either in the form of correctly combined vegetable proteins or animal proteins as above. Use unhulled sesame paste mixed with balsamic vinegar as a dressing to increase calcium intake.
- Soup with the addition of beans and grains, a little yoghurt or parmesan cheese.
- Any of the dinner choices or the breakfast energy drink.

Dinner ideas

Dinner should contain at least five different vegies, cooked or raw depending on season and preference; some protein; and a serve of complex carbohydrate like rice, root vegies, beans, or pasta.

To keep animal protein to a minimum, combine meat with grain or bean dishes. Examples might be lamb and chickpea casserole, or similar combination, common in the Middle East and the south-eastern European countries; pasta and tomato sauce with tuna; stir-fry vegetables with a little meat, and served with rice, common in Asia. Or:

- Steamed vegetables with rice and tofu.
- Stir-fry beef and vegetables with rice.
- Steamed vegetables with lentils and rice.
- Grilled or baked fish with vegetables or salad.
- Minestrone soup with beans and parmesan cheese.

Snacks
Choose high-calcium snacks such as dried figs, almonds, unhulled sesame seed paste on a dry biscuit, or yoghurt.

Fluids
- Limit caffeine-containing beverages to two cups of coffee or four cups of tea (and you know that doesn't mean you can have two megajolt triple caffeine-screaming long blacks).
- Drink at least 2 litres of water daily.

FOOD FOR HEALING

In the past decade, the belief that diet can improve health and reduce the risk of a number of serious diseases has become proven fact. In particular, a low-fat diet reduces the risk of cancer and heart disease. And a diet high in fibre and plant oestrogens is likely to reduce your risk of getting oestrogen-dependent cancers such as breast cancer.

Short-term therapeutic diets can be designed with a specific outcome in mind like getting rid of a complaint, or long-term diets might have a preventative focus. A diet might be designed around a specific life event such as breastfeeding, becoming menopausal or needing surgery.

Therapeutic diets

Be sure to get a professional diagnosis before trying any therapeutic diets designed for specific complaints. This is a serious business and you don't want to go faffing about with de-tox diets or the like without knowing exactly what you want to achieve and why. Stop when you get the required result.

 ## Continuing functional hypoglycaemia diet

© copyright Ruth Trickey

To be supervised by your health practitioner

When your symptoms have stopped, you can try coming off and following the 20 Diet Hints listed earlier in this chapter.

Functional hypoglycaemia is caused by fluctuations in the blood sugar levels. Symptoms include fatigue, lethargy, sleepiness, insomnia, irritability, weakness, headache, sugar cravings or unusual hunger. This syndrome is most likely to happen after stress, or the consumption of excess sugars and highly refined foods. If you have PMS or menstrual migraines, this diet is likely to help.

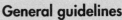

General guidelines

- Eat small amounts of protein regularly at meals and with snacks.
- Eat small meals often.
- Avoid all sugar, honey and dried fruit.
- Consume only small quantities of unsweetened, diluted fruit juice.
- Avoid all stimulants such as tea, coffee, chocolate, and cola drinks.
- Avoid alcohol and cigarettes.
- Eat wholegrain foods; avoid white flour and refined cereals.
- *Always* eat breakfast.

Protein

All animal protein is 'complete', and therefore meals containing milk products, eggs, meat or fish provide first class protein. Incomplete (plant) protein foods, however, need to be combined with complementary foods and eaten at the same meal to provide the same quality protein as animal protein.

Eat beans with grains: tofu (from soya beans) and rice; lentils and rice; corn and beans; buckwheat and tempeh; muesli and soya milk; kidney beans and barley. Or eat beans with seeds: tahini and beans; tofu and sesame seeds.

Or eat grains with nuts: nut butters on bread; rice and cashews; rice and peanut sauce.

Suggested menus

Breakfast
Choose from:

- Fruit with yoghurt, seeds and ground almonds.

- Wholegrain bread toast with nut butters, hommos or egg.

- Home-made muesli: oats, rolled barley, rice flakes, rice bran, seeds, coconut, and crushed almonds or cashews. Add fresh fruit and soya milk, low-fat milk or yoghurt as desired.

- Cooked cereal: oats (porridge), rice or buck-wheat, with a selection of seeds.

Morning, afternoon or supper snack
Choose from:

- A small handful of mixed seeds and nuts.

- Half a banana and a small handful of almonds.

- A glass of soya milk with seeds and nuts

- A small container of low-fat yoghurt.

- Two wholegrain dry biscuits with nut butters or hommos.

- Energy drink: Blend together half a cup of fresh fruit or juice, half a cup of low-fat yoghurt, and seeds with a small handful of almonds, and/or wheatgerm and lecithin.

Lunch

Choose from:

- Mixed vegetable salad with protein—either fish, cheese, hommos, meat or other appropriately combined vegetable proteins.
- Salad sandwich with protein as above.
- Vegetable soup with yoghurt, cheese, or a combination of beans and grains.
- One of the dinner choices.

Dinner

Choose from:

- Bean and grain dish: stir-fry vegies with rice and tofu; dhal with vegetables and rice; tortilla and beans; buckwheat noodles with vegetables and tempeh; vegetable soup with barley and red kidney beans.
- Grain and nut meal: steamed vegies with rice and peanut sauce; stir-fry vegies with cashew nuts; pasta and pesto sauce.
- Beans and seeds: many of the Middle Eastern vegetarian meals are based on the principle of combined vegie proteins, like felafel and hommos.
- Meat or fish with plenty of vegies.

Eat smaller meals than you usually do, but eat more often: six half-size meals should be substituted for three normal-size meals.

111

Continuing diet for irritable bowel syndrome

To be supervised by your health practitioner

When your symptoms have stopped, you can try coming off and following the 20 Diet Hints listed earlier in this chapter.

These dietary recommendations help to reduce the spasm, pain and bloating of irritable bowel syndrome, and to regulate bowel function.

Seed breakfast
The seed breakfast consists of a combination of seeds, pectin-containing fruit and yoghurt.

In summer
- Linseeds
- Almonds
- Pumpkin seeds
- Sesame seeds
- Sunflower seeds
- Rice bran

These seeds are ground daily (ground to a consistency of coarsely ground coffee) and then combined with the bran in quantities equal by weight. Any left-overs must always be refrigerated. Mix about 2 tablespoons of seed and bran mix with the following ingredients.

Plus, fruit:
- Grated raw apple *or*
- Stewed apple, pear or plums.
  Plus, yoghurt:
- Plain, (unsweetened) low-fat yoghurt with live cultures (Jalna, Lesna, Hakea and Hellenic are all good brands.)

Chuck it all in a bowl and dig in.

In winter
Cooked grains:
Add 2 tablespoons of the seed mix to porridge or rice after cooking and eat with warmed stewed fruit. Yoghurt can either be eaten with the fruit and grains or eaten as a side dish.

Herb tea
Melissa officinalis (lemon balm) *Matricaria recutita* (chamomile) and *Mentha piperita* (peppermint tea) in equal quantities are prepared as for ordinary tea (2 teaspoons per cup).
Dose: 1–2 cups between each meal.

Foods to avoid or reduce
- Stimulants such as tea, coffee and cola drinks.
- Cereals made from 100 per cent wheat bran.
- Fried food, pastry, cream and ice-cream.
- Breads and other foods with yeast.
- Refined sugar and foods containing refined sugars.
- Alcohol, especially beer and wine.

MINERALS

It is better to get all minerals from food, but if this isn't possible (as opposed to just inconvenient) you can take supplements. Always check with your health practitioner for acceptable doses for you.

Calcium

A consistently high calcium intake can improve bone density at all ages, prevent osteoporosis and fractures, and treat osteoporosis. The only exception is in the years immediately after menopause when the rapidly declining oestrogens exert a stronger effect. How long this lasts

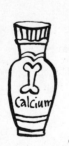

isn't entirely clear, but researchers think that it may be around five years and perhaps even up to ten years. Several years after menopause, calcium is again useful in reducing bone loss. Calcium supplements should contain magnesium because both minerals are required to improve bone density—calcium improves bone density while magnesium increases the rate of retention of calcium in the bone. (Dairy foods are not much chop as a lone source of calcium because of their low magnesium content.)

Menopausal women should consume two to three serves of low-fat dairy products per day combined with other foods that contain both calcium and magnesium: canned fish with edible bones such as salmon and sardines, and calcium-fortified soy milk are good examples.

Recommended daily allowance (RDA) for calcium

Infants	350–550 milligrams
Children aged 1–10 years	800 milligrams
Teenagers	1,200 milligrams
Young women 20–35 years	800–1000 milligrams
Pregnant/breastfeeding women	1500 milligrams
Premenopausal woman 35 years and over	1000 milligrams
Postmenopausal women	1500 milligrams
Women with low bone density	1500 milligrams

Types of calcium supplements

Calcium carbonate, the most commonly prescribed calcium supplement, is not usually well absorbed (as little as 4 per cent is taken up by those with low gastric acid and stomach acidity usually declines with age) and is of little value in improving bone density. Calcium citrate is useful for women with low gastric acid levels, and is generally thought to be a safe form of calcium to take over the long term. Calcium lactate and gluconate also have good absorption rates. In general, calcium absorption seems to be better when ingested with food, so supplements should be taken at meal times. Brekky is probably the easiest time to take your pills, but it is common for some doctors to recommend that you take calcium in the evening to offset the calcium loss that occurs overnight as a result of bed rest. Take them at the time when you are inclined to be most regular. Calcium supplements are also best taken in 500 milligrams doses so might need to be taken twice daily, depending on how much you're getting in your diet.

Guidelines for supplementing with calcium

Every woman, regardless of age, should assess the amount of calcium in her diet. If your intake is below the recommended level, you should take a supplement to make up the difference. To assess your intake, you can keep a record of all foods eaten over a week. The approximate level of calcium is then calculated by using the list on page 118) which gives levels of calcium per 100 grams of food. Total daily calcium intakes are added together and divided by the number of days the diary has been kept to get an average daily intake. To take an obvious example, if your recommended daily intake is 1000 milligrams and your average daily intake is only 800 milligrams, you should take a 200 milligrams supplement of calcium.

What is 'elemental' calcium (and magnesium)?

All mineral supplements have an 'elemental' figure on their label. For example, 1050 milligrams of calcium citrate has 250 milligrams of elemental calcium. The 'elemental' figure is the amount of the actual mineral in the preparation. The remaining 800 milligrams is the weight of the other stuff (in this case citrate). The table below shows the 'elemental' amounts for some common calcium and magnesium supplements:

Calcium citrate	1050 milligrams
elemental calcium	250 milligrams
Calcium hydroxyapatite	1000 milligrams
elemental calcium	240 milligrams
Calcium orotate	1000 milligrams
elemental calcium	100 milligrams
Magnesium aspartate	1000 milligrams
elemental magnesium	80 milligrams
Magnesium orotate	800 milligrams
elemental magnesium	52 milligrams

Low-kilojoule calcium sources
Women with heart disease, diabetes, or who are overweight, should consider these low-fat sources. All these low-kilojoule food sources have 300 milligrams of calcium:

$1\frac{1}{4}$ cups of cooked spinach or other greens
2 cups cooked broccoli
1 cup Physical milk
1 cup plain low-fat yoghurt
$\frac{1}{4}$ cup grated parmesan
50 grams Swiss or cheddar cheese
$1\frac{1}{2}$ cups whole milk
$1\frac{1}{4}$ cups plain yoghurt
200 grams tofu
1 can sardines
300 grams tinned salmon
2 cups low-fat cottage cheese

Good sources of calcium

This chart shows how many milligrams of calcium are in 100 grams of food.

Dairy products

Skim milk powder (dry)	1190	Goat's milk	130
Whole milk powder (dry)	900	Skimmed cow's milk	123
Whey powder	645	Buttermilk	115
Physical milk 100 ml	205	Cow's milk whole	115
Yoghurt—cow's	180	Human milk	30
Rev milk 100 ml	150		

Cheese

Parmesan	1091	Camembert (30% fat)	600
Gruyere	1000	Danish Blue	580
Mozzarella	817	Blue (50% fat)	540
Cheddar	810	Camembert (60%fat)	400
Gouda	810	Fetta	353
Edam (30% fat)	800	Ricotta	223
Edam (45% fat)	678	Cottage (low-fat)	77
Gorgonzola	612	Cottage	67

Eggs   56

Fish

Whitebait	860	Scallops	120
Sardines (canned)	550	Salmon (canned)	100

Soya products

Soya milk (dry)	330	Tofu	170
Soya grits	255	So Good soy milk	116
Dried soya beans	225	Vita Soy soy milk	32
Soya flour, full fat	210		

Nuts

Almonds	250	Walnuts	60
Brazil	180	Macadamia	50
Pistachio	136	Hazelnuts	45
Pecan	75	Peanut butter	35
Peanuts (fresh)	60	Cashews	30

Seeds

Unhulled sesame seeds	1160	Sunflower seeds	98
Linseeds	271	Pumpkin seeds	52
Hulled sesame seeds	110		

Grains and cereals

White flour	350	Wheat germ	69
Muesli (depends on brand)	200	Wheat crispbread	60
Wheat flour (white or brown)	150	Porridge	55
Wheat bran	110	Rye crispbread	50
Bread (brown or white)	100	Brown rice	33
All Bran	75	Weetbix	33
Rice bran	69		

Meat 10–20

Legumes (cooked)

Navy beans	95	Lentils	50
Chickpeas	70	Black-eyed beans	40
Kidney beans	70	Split peas	22

Sprouts

Alfalfa sprouts	28	Lentil sprouts	12
Mung bean sprouts	20		

Vegetables

Parsley	260	Onions	135
Watercress	190	Spinach	135
Dandelion greens	185	Broccoli	125
Spring onions	140	Silverbeet	115

Fruits

Dried figs	260	Rhubarb (stewed)	93
Lemons	110	Orange juice (100 ml)	60
Lemon juice (100 ml)	8	Blackberries	60
Other fruit except dried	10–50		

Other

Kelp	1095	Carob powder	355
Crude molasses	654	Brewers' yeast	210
Torula yeast	425		

Other minerals involved in bone metabolism

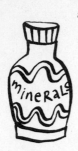

Apart from calcium, a number of other minerals are important for maintaining good bone density. The most important are magnesium, phosphorus, zinc and boron. Magnesium and zinc are covered in full in the following sections, but phosphorus and boron we look at here, as well as some of the other trace minerals and vitamins necessary for bone health.

Phosphorus is needed by every cell in the body for energy production, and is essential for the health of bones and teeth. High intakes are common because they're found in meat and high concentrations are in soft drinks. The recommended daily intake of 800 milligrams per day (US RDA 1980) is easily achieved or exceeded. Too much phosphorus and not enough calcium can increase calcium loss from bone.

Boron, while sounding like a local on Planet Zorg, is actually a trace mineral which seems to affect the synthesis of the active form of oestrogen and vitamin D in the body. It seems to have an oestrogen-like effect and there is some suggestion that boron deficiency reduces the positive effects of HRT on bone density and other symptoms of oestrogen deficiency during the menopause.

Fruits, vegetables and nuts are the main sources of boron. Animal proteins are not a good source. The best hits of it are found in prunes, almonds and raisins, which contain approximately 2.5 milligrams per 100 grams of food, and wine which contains 0.8 milligrams per 100 millilitres glass. Other rich sources include parsley, dates, hazelnuts, peanuts, apples and peaches. Boron is now also available in some supplements designed specifically to improve bone density. The recommended daily allowance is between 1 and 10 milligrams of boron daily.

Manganese, **copper**, **silicon** and **strontium** are the other minerals important to bone health. They are involved in collagen synthesis and in the processes of bone mineralisation. Manganese, copper and zinc supplements have been shown to improve bone weakness when levels of these minerals are low in the blood. Strontium deficiency also causes problems with bone and collagen synthesis. All of these minerals are found in trace levels in foods, particularly of plant origin, and eating a wide variety of different fruits and vegetables is usually sufficient to prevent deficiency.

Silicon is another of the important nutrients for the health of collagen tissue. It is a vital cross-linking agent that contributes to the structure and resilience of connective tissue. As well, it is involved in bone calcification, making it an essential mineral for bone health. It is available in a wide variety of vegetables and so deficiency is rarely a problem.

Assimilation and absorption

Eating sensible amounts regularly, eating slowly and chewing food well all aid assimilation of minerals. If you get symptoms of bloating, dyspepsia and indigestion you may have poor gastric acid secretion which impairs absorption of calcium salts. When gastric acid levels are low, calcium supplements must always be taken with food as this tends to normalise absorption. Stimulating gastric secretions by eating bitter and sour foods can also improve uptake of minerals.

Diarrhoea

Diarrhoea has already been mentioned as a risk factor for osteoporosis. The causes of diarrhoea should be identified and treated promptly. One teaspoon of slippery elm powder two or three times each day can be useful.

Vitamins

Apart from vitamin D, the main role for vitamins in bone health is in the protection and maintenance of collagen. Vitamins B6, B12, A, C, E, K and folic acid are all essential. Vitamin D, from sunlight and the diet, contributes

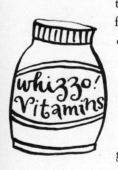

to improved bone density. Researchers have found that high percentages of women with osteoporosis are vitamin D deficient, thought to be because they work or stay indoors all day. Try getting a little sunshine every day, preferably when UV levels are lowest in the mornings or later in the afternoon. A good multivitamin supplement, or better still, a good diet should cover these factors for you.

Phyto-oestrogens

There is a suggestion that phyto-oestrogens may have positive effects on bone density. As yet, the research is in its early stages, but there is growing evidence to support the contention that a high daily intake may prevent bone density loss. Some soy-related supplements such as ipri-flavone, are also showing promise in improving bone density.

Magnesium

Magnesium is crucial in the mix, because osteoporosis is associated with lower than normal bone magnesium levels and because it increases calcium absorption from food, enhances calcium retention in the body, and increases bone density. Despite this, look out: medically prescribed supplements rarely contain magnesium.

The RDA for magnesium is 400–800 milligrams a day and should equal about half the calcium intake. For example, if you've been through the menopause and have a daily calcium intake of 1500 milligrams , make sure you also get 800 milligrams of magnesium.

Bones

Magnesium is almost as important for bone health as calcium. As we've already said, it improves the absorption of calcium from food and increases its retention in the body. A high intake of calcium inhibits the absorption of magnesium. Foods traditionally thought of as being useful for bone density, such as dairy products, are also relatively low in magnesium (a cup of milk contains 290 milligrams of calcium, but only 35 milligrams of magnesium) which raises doubts about the suitability of large intakes of dairy products for bone health. Magnesium, either alone or with calcium, offsets the usual overnight bone mineral loss.

The heart
Magnesium protects the heart muscle from getting overexcited which can cause irregularities in the heart beat.

PMS
Magnesium and vitamin B6 can help alter the hormone levels and protect against PMS.

Signs and symptoms of magnesium deficiency
Weakness and/or tiredness; poor muscle co-ordination; muscle cramps; grimaces, tremors of the tongue, 'flickering' eyelids; premenstrual symptoms; apathy; insomnia, hyperactivity; susceptibility to toxic effects of the drug digoxin; abnormalities of the heart's rhythm, an abnormal reading on an electrocardiograph (ECG) which traces heart activity; loss of appetite, nausea, constipation; confusion, disorientation and memory impairment, learning disabilities; vertigo; difficulty swallowing or throat constriction.

Obviously these symptoms can have other serious causes, but when no obvious cause can be found, improved magnesium intake may help.

Recommended daily allowance
The recommended daily intake for magnesium is 400–800 milligrams for women.

Good sources of magnesium

This chart shows how many milligrams of magnesium are in 100 grams of food.

Grains

Wheat bran*	520	Wheat germ	300
Whole wheat flour	140	Porridge	110
Muesli	100	Rye flour	92
White flour	36		

Seafood

Prawns	110

Vegetables

Beet tops	106	Silverbeet	65
Spinach	59	Raw parsley	52
Beans	35	Green peas	33
Broccoli	24	Beetroot	23

Beans and nuts

Brazil nuts	410	Soya flour	290
Almonds	260	Peanuts	180
Walnuts	130		

Fruits

Dried figs	92	Dried apricots	65
Avocado	30	Banana	20
Grapefruit juice	18		

---

* Foods that are rich in magnesium, such as bran, may not provide the best source of minerals. Magnesium can become bound to the phytates in bran which reduce absorption. Whole foods from a wide variety of sources is the best way to attain a good intake of easily absorbed magnesium.

Zinc

Most women don't get enough zinc. Zinc is essential for collagen health, normal bone development, and the normal functioning of vitamin D. A recent Australian survey revealed that 85 per cent of women were receiving less than the recommended daily allowance for zinc. Zinc levels are lower in elderly people with osteoporosis.

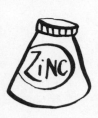 Manganese is required for bone mineralisation and the synthesis of collagen in bone and has been found to be deficient in osteoporotic women. When zinc, manganese and copper were added to a calcium supplement, postmenopausal bone loss slowed more than with calcium alone.

Some possible symptoms of zinc deficiency

Slow growth; infertility/delayed sexual maturation; hair loss; skin conditions of various kinds; diarrhoea; immune deficiencies; behavioural and sleep disturbances; night blindness; impaired taste and smell; white spots on fingernails; delayed wound healing; post-op complications; dandruff; impaired glucose tolerance; connective tissue disease; reduced appetite.

Zinc deficiency can be caused by

Anorexia nervosa, fad diets, 'weight-loss' diets; exclusion diets for food allergies; a strict vegetarian diet; restricted protein diets; long-term intravenous therapy or tube feeding through the nose; alcoholism.

Zinc absorption may be hampered by
High-fibre diets; iron tablets; coeliac disease (gluten intolerance); food allergies; low or absent gastric acid levels; alcoholic cirrhosis; a dicky pancreas.

You need extra zinc if you're
- going through puberty or a growth spurt
- pregnant or breastfeeding
- taking diuretics
- on the drug penicillamine, a detoxifying drug
- suffering from psoriasis, exfoliative dermatitis, or excessive sweating
- troubled by intestinal parasites or hookworm
- drinking too much grog
- suffering from liver disease including viral hepatitis
- prone to chronic diarrhoea and ileostomy fluid loss
- recovering from surgery or trauma
- diagnosed with cancer

Recommended daily allowance
12–15 milligrams a day for women.

Good sources of zinc
This chart shows how many milligrams of zinc are in 100 grams of food.

Fresh oysters (as if you'd be having those everyday)	45–75	Peanuts	3
		Sardines	3
Dark chicken meat	2.85	Hazelnuts	3.5
Wheat bran	16	Walnuts	2.25
Wheat germ	13	Wholewheat bread	1.65
Dried ginger root	7	Prawns	1.15

Continued over page

127

Zinc sources continued

Brazil nuts	7	Whole egg	1.10
Red meats	4.5–8.5	Non-fat cow milk	0.75
Parmesan cheese	4	Porridge	0.5
Dried peas	4	Raw carrots	0.5

Iron

Iron requirements for women are around 80 per cent higher than for men. It is estimated that iron deficiency is the most common nutritional disease worldwide and that more than half of all women consume less than the recommended amount of 10–15 milligrams a day.

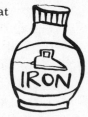

Those at most risk of iron deficiency

Pregnant women; women with heavy periods; children; vegetarians; serial dieters; people on strict exclusion diets; people with low gastric acid levels, such as after stomach surgery and with ageing; people with malnutrition. Iron deficiency is much less likely to be a problem after menopause, but during the peri-menopausal years when heavy periods can be a problem, many women become anaemic.

Iron deficiency or anaemia?

Iron is stored in the body in red blood cells, the liver, bone marrow, spleen, muscles and in the serum. A test for anaemia will determine only whether there is a depletion of iron stored in the red blood cells (the haemoglobin level), but not whether iron levels are high enough in the rest of the body.

The symptoms of iron deficiency can happen before

the red blood cells become depleted of iron. Many people are iron deficient even though their haemoglobin is normal. For this reason, many doctors now order a blood test to check iron stores in the plasma as well as the haemoglobin levels.

Symptoms of anaemia
Red blood cells need iron to be able to carry oxygen around the body. When that isn't around, anaemia symptoms happen, including poor stamina; shortness of breath on exertion; unreasonable limb fatigue and dizziness. Other symptoms seem to be related to the lack of iron in the serum, called iron deficiency.

Symptoms of iron deficiency
A red sore tongue and cracks in the corners of the mouth; excess hair loss; concave finger nails; reduced resistance to infection; poor digestion caused by low gastric acid levels. (Iron deficiency can cause decreased production of gastric acid and can be caused by it—a vicious circle.) Some people with iron deficiency have a strong desire to chew ice. In children, symptoms include not thriving; slow learning; reduced infection resistance and poor appetite.

How to improve iron absorption
Apart from increasing the amount of available iron in the diet, there are a number of other ways to increase iron levels:
- Eat vitamin C rich foods, particularly when consuming foods high in iron.

- Add acidic dressings, such as lemon juice and vinegar, to iron-rich foods. This is a common southern Mediterranean practice, where there is a high incidence of inherited anaemia and the traditional diet contains little red meat.
- Eat bitter vegetables or fruit before or during the meal to increase the flow of gastric acid which will in turn improve the absorption of minerals. Alcoholic aperitifs, grapefruit, Swedish bitters and bitter green vegetables can all be used. Bitter vegetables are best because they usually contain iron as well as stimulating its absorption.
- When low gastric acid levels are accompanied by iron deficiency, taking iron may improve both.
- Avoid tea (especially black tea) or coffee until the iron deficiency improves. The tannin in tea binds with iron, making it difficult to absorb.
- Coffee also reduces absorption, especially if taken with or after a meal, but not when taken more than one hour before eating.
- Definitely don't take iron tablets with a cup of tea or coffee.

Diagnosing low iron stores
Iron deficiency causes the symptoms described above and should respond to a low-dose iron supplement within a few weeks. Iron should not be taken unnecessarily as it will accumulate in the body and may become toxic. If symptoms do not respond, seek advice and ask for a blood test which evaluates serum iron levels.

Recommended daily allowance
10–15 milligrams a day for women.

Good sources of iron
This chart shows how many milligrams of iron are in 100 grams of food.

Meat, fish and eggs
Mussels	7.7	Oysters	6.0
Lean beef	3.4	Lean lamb	2.7
Sardines	2.4	Eggs	2.0
Dark chicken meat	1.9	Lean pork	1.3
Light chicken meat	0.6	Cod	0.4

Grains
Special K	20.0	Wheat bran	12.9
AllBran	12.0	Wheat germ	10.0
Soyaflour	9.1	Weetbix	7.6
Raw oatmeal	4.1	Whole wheat flour	4.0
Rye biscuits	3.7	Whole wheat bread	2.5
White bread	1.7		

Legumes and vegetables
Raw parsley	8.0	Spinach	3.4
Silverbeet	3.0	Haricot beans	2.5
Lentils	2.4	Leeks	2.0
Spring onions	1.2	Peas	1.2
Broccoli	1.0	Raw mushrooms	1.0
Lettuce	0.9	Jacket potatoes	0.6

Fruits
Dried peaches	6.8	Dried figs	4.2
Dried apricots	4.1	Prunes	2.9
Sultanas	1.8	Currants	1.8
Raisins	1.6	Dates	1.6
Avocado	1.5	Stewed prunes	1.4
Raspberries	1.2	Fresh apricots	0.4

Continued over page

Other

Yeast	20.0	Almonds	4.2
Brazil nuts	2.8	Walnuts	2.4
Peanuts	2.0	Hazelnuts	1.1

PLANT OESTROGENS

What? Not more oestrogens! The oestrogens made in our bodies are called endogenous oestrogens. Some plants naturally contain components that are structurally similar to oestrogen and can have similar effects on the body. These are called plant oestrogens. They are also known as phyto-oestrogens. (Pronounced fight-oh-east-roe-jens.)

Eating some phyto-oestrogens every day is a good idea. Basically, they're thought to be protective against cancer, and they may also reduce the incidence of oestrogen-responsive diseases such as endometriosis and fibroids. Extra amounts can help stop menopausal hot flushes.

Positive research results are relevant for just eating phyto-oestrogens as part of a normal diet—there is no evidence to support getting into complicated regimes of weighing foods and taking long-term supplements.

The simple message of this section is to whack into your diet some more phyto-oestrogens found in soya stuff, legumes, sprouty things and linseeds. Here's why.

What are phyto-oestrogens?

One of the first hints that hormones in plants could affect mammals came from the discovery that infertile sheep had been eating clover containing 'plant oestrogens'. Now, don't panic. This doesn't mean that if you eat clover-based honey you're infertile, or anything like that. If you've been going through a paddock or two of clover every week you might need to worry. (In more ways than one.)

Anyway, what we do now know, after researchers have ferreted around in laboratories, and a bit of trial and error, is that plant oestrogens are found in lots of growing things and that eating them can affect human health. In the way of scientists, they found a whizzbangery scientific term for plants containing oestrogenic components —the word is phyto-oestrogen, meaning a plant containing an oestrogen-like substance. (*Phyto* is Greek for plant.)

Phyto-oestrogens we eat that can affect our health include isoflavonoids, coumestans and lignans; the triterpenoid and steroidal saponins, the phytosterols and the resorcylic acid lactones, including zearalenone. All of them are naturally occurring compounds found in a large range of whole foods including grains, seeds (linseeds have lots of phyto-oestrogens but linseed oil doesn't, for example), legumes, and medicinal plants, as well as other common foods.

Foods with plant oestrogens

Isoflavones: especially soya beans and all other legumes; whole grains.

Coumestans: especially soya sprouts; and all other sprouted beans or legumes, split peas, mung beans.

Lignans: especially linseeds; and whole rye, buckwheat, millet, sesame and sunflower seeds, legumes and beans, whole grains.

Resorcylic acid lactones: oats, barley, rye, sesame seeds, wheat, and peas.

Steroidal saponins: especially real liquorice, and potato.

The effects of phyto-oestrogens

The effects of plant oestrogens on our hormones are pretty complicated. They can cause periods to get lighter and less frequent, reduce the incidence of oestrogen-dependent cancers, and help with menopausal symptoms, especially hot flushes.

Asian women who eat a traditional diet excrete higher amounts of endogenous oestrogen than women who eat a 'Western' diet, which some researchers believe accounts for their lower risk of breast cancer. Soya products consumed regularly in Asian countries contain high levels of phyto-oestrogens, and are said to be responsible for these positive effects, along with genes.

The lignans and some of the isoflavones require normal levels of bowel bacteria to turn them into the right stuff, so if you've taken, or are taking antibiotics, you probably won't get the full benefit. Yoghurt seems to help maintain the right bacteria.

How they work

Phyto-oestrogens share many of the same biological roles with oestrogens produced in the body. This is probably because phyto-oestrogens and body-made oestrogens are structurally similar, and both have the ability to interact with oestrogen receptors. We seem to need the phyto-oestrogens to balance our levels of oestrogens produced in the body throughout life.

According to lab tests, the oestrogenic effect of a phyto-oestrogen is from 160 to many thousands of times weaker than the body-made oestrogen oestradiol (pronounced eastro-die-al).

Before the menopause

Before menopause, the phyto-oestrogens we eat may help to protect against the 'proliferative effects' of too much oestrogen and reduce the incidence of related diseases like breast cancer, endometriosis and fibroids.

Some diseases and cancers may develop because of the overstimulating effect of too much oestrogen, but it's possible for phyto-oestrogens to prevent many of the more stimulatory oestrogens from occupying receptor sites: this is called competitive inhibition. Competitive inhibition is believed to be one of the ways that diets rich in isoflavonoids and lignans reduce the risk of oestrogen-dependent cancers. Tamoxifen, a drug which is used to treat breast cancer, is structurally related to the phyto-oestrogens.

The phyto-oestrogens are also capable of slowing down the production of extra, non-ovarian oestrogen produced in the fat tissues. As we've said, eating more soya products seems to lower the risk of breast cancer. This may be related to the phyto-oestrogens or be a result of many compounds acting together. There is evidence that eating phyto-oestrogens can help *prevent* cancer, but it isn't yet known whether eating phyto-oestrogens will help you if you already have an oestrogen-responsive breast cancer.

The isoflavonoids and lignans also stimulate liver production of sex hormone binding globulin (SHBG).

SHBG binds to the sex hormones, especially androgens and oestrogens, and acts as a carrier protein. When the major portion of these hormones are bound to SHBG in the blood, they are less available to bind to hormone-sensitive tissues. This is believed to be another way in which phyto-oestrogens lower the incidence of hormone-related diseases.

Period regulation
Other more immediate benefits from phyto-oestrogens include lighter periods and longer menstrual cycles. They also reduce the risk of endometrial hyperplasia (too much cell production in the uterine lining), which is a pre-cancerous condition.

Improved bone density?
There is a suggestion that phyto-oestrogens may have positive effects on bone density. As yet, the research is in its early stages, but there is evidence to support the contention that a high daily intake may prevent bone density loss. Some soy-related supplements such as ipri-flavone, are also showing promise in improving bone density.

After menopause
After menopause, the phyto-oestrogens have a mildly oestrogenic effect because they become more prevalent in a relatively oestrogen-poor environment.

Recently Australian researchers found soya flour (high in phyto-oestrogens) decreased hot flushes by 40 per cent compared to 25 per cent in a wheat flour group (lower in phyto-oestrogens). Other studies have shown that phyto-oestrogens consumed from whole foods such as soybeans can lower both cholesterol and blood pressure.

Getting your phyto-oestrogens

Increasing soya intake can be as easy as substituting low-fat soy milk for ordinary milk and using soya flour in cooking. Tofu is very useful, and even 100 grams a day can reduce hot flushes and vaginal dryness. Dried or 'fresh' soya beans (you can buy them frozen in Asian food shops) can be added to soups and bean dishes. As little as 25 grams or about 2 heaped dessertspoons of ground linseeds per day can help to reduce symptoms of low oestrogen levels, including vaginal dryness. Linseeds contain lignans and can be used in cooking or ground and added to muesli, porridge, or drinks, like a smoothie. (The easiest way to grind seeds is in a coffee grinder you don't use for coffee beans. It's best to grind and eat them immediately so there's no chance of rancidity.)

What Now?

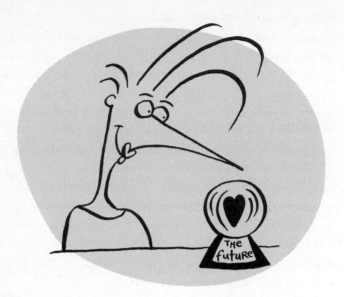

BOOKS

A Guide to Menopause, Dr Deborah Saltman, Choice Magazine Publishing. Topics include HRT, alternative therapies, osteoporosis, sexuality and web contacts. The Australian Consumers Association has a mail order service on 02 9577 3399.

The Change by Germaine Greer, Penguin Books Australia, 1993. A typically singular look at the menopause by a post-menopausal expatriate Australian intellectual feminist icon.

The Curse by Karen Houppert, Allen & Unwin, Sydney, 1999. An informative and political examination of how women are taught to be ashamed and secretive about periods. If you have a lot of trouble with periods you may quarrel with the 'periods are natural and wonderful' message but it's still a fascinating story about 'the last unmentionable taboo: menstruation' and the surprisingly long-lasting theme of 'feminine hygiene'.

WEBSITES

Use your search engine to search for websites using key words like *menopause* or *early menopause*. If you don't have access to the World Wide Web through a home computer, try your local library or internet café. (If you turn off the picture function, the downloading of words from a website will speed up and therefore be cheaper.)

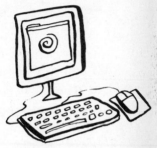

www.menopause.org
The website of the North American Menopause Society, 'the leading scientific nonprofit organization devoted to promoting women's health during midlife and beyond through an understanding of menopause' run by health professionals in the field. Covers peri-menopause, early menopause, symptoms and solutions, suggested reading, news, medical and other advances and a member's site — are all available on this comprehensive website.

www.mum.org
The Museum of Menstruation and Women's Health

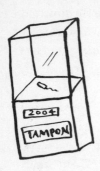

Okay, it's pretty weird that a guy has set this up and dedicated it to 'Mom' but it's full of amazing facts about the history of periods, euphemisms, books about the subject, practical and impractical products used to deal with periods, attitudes through the ages and chat rooms. Includes a page about the cats that live in the real museum of menstruation in Washington DC, but a fun, if odd visit can be had on the net.

www.menopause-online.com
If you can't find it on this site, it never existed. A link to 9 million medical articles on menopause, live chat room, and approximately 678 gerzillion specific info-based items on everything from what Oprah Winfrey says about testosterone to arthritis, HRT, herbs and dealing with memory problems.

www.menopause.org.au
Australasian Menopause Society
PO Box 876
Kingsford NSW 2032
Phone: 02 9382 6732
Fax: 02 9382 6728
Email: ams@netlink.com.au
There are over 2 million post-menopausal women in Australia, and every year about 80,000 new women join this group. These women constitute 40% of all health

care visits in Australia. This organisation is made up of doctors and other professionals in the area of menopause and includes contacts for clinics in Australia, and, somewhat mysteriously, Peru and Switzerland. A number of pamphlets on menopause management are available.

www.awhn.org.au
Australian Women's Health Network
Women's health advocacy network run by volunteers which lobby the government and try to post important and useful links and information on many women's health subjects. Go to the Women's Health Issues link on their home page and click on your area of interest.

EARLY MENOPAUSE

The Premature Menopause Book by Kathryn Petras, Wholecare, 1999. Includes signs and symptoms, which tests to ask your doctor for, and importantly, the emotional as well as medical implications. Covers alternatives to natural fertility, and recommends HRT for women with premature menopause. American, with US info and support groups.

The Monash Medical Centre in Melbourne has an Early Menopause Clinic, phone 03 9594 6666.

www.earlymenopause.com
Support, resources, treatment, news.

SUPPORT GROUPS

The following contact points can be used to find specific support groups for your illness, information and advice and for various contacts in your area. These groups nearly always have their funding cut, so you can help out by ringing your local politician to say we need them properly funded.

Women's Information Services

These groups will be able to point you in any direction you need. They're a clearing house for any requests for information.

Australian Capital Territory
Women's Information and Referral Centre
Level 6, 197 London Circuit
Canberra City ACT 2600
Phone: 02 6205 1075, 02 6205 1076
Fax: 02 6205 1077
Email: wirc@act.gov.au
Homepage: www.wirc.act.gov.au

New South Wales
Women's Information and Referral Service
Department for Women
Level 4, 181 Castlereagh Street
Sydney NSW 2000
Phone: 02 9287 1810, 1800 817 227
Fax: 02 9287 1823
Email: dfw@women.nsw.gov.au
Homepage: www.women.nsw.gov.au

Northern Territory

Darwin
Women's Health Strategy Unit
Department of Health and Community Services
PO Box 40596
Casuarina NT 0811
Phone: 08 8999 2804

Alice Springs
Women's Information Centre
Ground floor, Eurilpa House, Todd Mall
Alice Springs NT 0870
PO Box 721, Alice Springs NT 0871
Phone: 08 8951 5880
Fax: 08 8951 5884
Email: wicalice.ths@nt.gov.au

Queensland

Brisbane
Women's Info Link
56 Mary Street
Brisbane QLD 4000
PO Box 185, Albert Street, Brisbane QLD 4002
Phone: 07 3224 2211, 1800 177 577
Fax: 1800 656 122
Email: infolink@premiers.qld.gov.au
Homepage: www.qldwoman.qld.gov.au

Cairns
Women's Information and Referral Centre
230 Mulgrave Road
Cairns QLD 4870
Phone: 07 4051 9366
Fax: 07 4031 6750
Email: wirc@wirc.org.au

South Australia
Women's Information Service
136 North Terrace, Station Arcade
Adelaide SA 5000
Phone: 08 8303 0590, 1800 188 158
Fax: 08 8303 0576
Email: info@wif.sa.gov.au
Homepage: www.wif.sa.gov.au

Tasmania
Women Tasmania
140-142 Macquarie Street
Hobart TAS 7000
Phone: 03 6233 2208, 1800 001 377
Fax: 03 6233 8833
Email: wt.admin@dpac.tas.gov.au
Homepage: www.women.tas.gov.au

Victoria
Women's Information and Referral Exchange
1st floor, 247 Flinders Lane
Melbourne VIC 3000
Phone: 03 9206 0870, 1300 134 130

Fax: 03 9654 6831
Email: wire@wire.org.au
Homepage: www.wire.org.au

Western Australia
Women's Information Service
1st floor, 141 St George's Terrace
Perth WA 6000
Phone: 08 9264 1900, 1800 199 174
Fax: 08 9264 1925
Email: wpo@dcd.wa.gov.au
Homepage: www.wa.gov.au/wpdo

Family Planning Clinics
For information on general women's health and screening
matters as well as contraception and pregnancy termination, you can't go past the Family Planning Clinics. Here
are their head offices. Phone for a service nearer you.

Australian Capital Territory
Health Promotion Centre
Childers Street
Canberra ACT 2600
GPO Box 1317
Canberra City ACT 2601
Phone: 02 6247 3077
Fax: 02 6257 5710
Email: fpact@familyplanningact.org.au
Homepage: www.familyplanningact.org.au

New South Wales
FPA Health
328-336 Liverpool Road
Ashfield NSW 2131
Phone: 02 8752 4300, 1300 658 886
Fax: 02 9716 6164
Email: enquiries@fpahealth.org.au
Homepage: www.fpahealth.org.au

Northern Territory
Family Planning Welfare
The Clock Tower, Unit 2
Dickward Drive
Coconut Grove NT 0810
Phone: 08 8948 0144
Fax: 08 8948 0626

Queensland
Family Planning Queensland (FPQ)
100 Alfred Street
Fortitude Valley QLD 4006
Phone: 07 3250 0200
Fax: 07 3854 1277
Homepage: www.fpq.asn.au

South Australia
Shine SA
17 Phillips Street
Kensington SA 5068
Phone: 08 8431 5177, 1800 188 171
Fax: 08 8364 2389
Homepage: www.shinesa.org.au

Tasmania
Family Planning Tasmania Inc.
2 Midwood Street
New Town TAS 7008
Phone: 03 6228 5244, 1800 007 119
Email: FamPlan.Hobt@tassie.net.au
Homepage: www.tased.edu.au/tasonline/sexedfpt

Victoria
Family Planning Victoria
901 Whitehorse Road
Box Hill VIC 3128
Phone: 03 9257 0100, 1800 013 952
Fax: 03 9257 0112
Email: fpv@fpv.org.au
Homepage: www.sexlife.com

Western Australia
Family Planning Western Australia (FPWA)
70 Roe Street
Northbridge WA 6003
Phone: 08 9227 6177, 1800 198 205
Fax: 08 9227 6871
Email: sexhelp@fpwa-health.org.au
Homepage: www.fpwa-health.org.au

HEALTH CARE CENTRES

For help in locating services and finding support groups and information about medical conditions. Call the relevant numbers to find local contacts in your suburb, district or town.

Australian Capital Territory
Women's Health Service
Corner Moore and Alinga Streets
Canberra City ACT 2601
Phone: 02 6205 1078
Fax: 02 6207 0143
Email: womens.health@act.gov.au

New South Wales
Women's Medical Centre
Suite 10 and 11, level 2
193 Macquarie Street
Sydney NSW 2000
Phone: 02 9231 2366
Fax: 02 9233 1020
Homepage: www.womensmedicalcentre.com

Northern Territory
Royal Darwin Hospital
Rockland Drive
Tiwi NT 0810
Phone: 08 8922 8888
Fax: 08 8922 8286
Homepage:
www.nt.gov.au/nths/royaldarwinhospital/welcome.htm

Queensland
Women's Health Queensland Wide
165 Gregory Terrace
Springhill QLD 4000
Phone: 07 3839 9962, 1800 017 676
Fax: 07 3831 7214
Email: whcb@womhealth.org.au
Homepage: www.womhealth.org.au

South Australia
Women's Health Statewide
64 Pennington Terrace
North Adelaide SA 5006
Phone: 08 8239 9600, 1800 182 098
Fax: 08 8239 9696
Email: info@whs.sa.gov.au
Homepage: www.whs.sa.gov.au

Tasmania
Hobart Women's Health Centre
326 Elizabeth Street
North Hobart TAS 7000
Phone: 03 6231 3212, 1800 353212
Fax: 03 6236 9449
Email: hwhc@trump.net.au
Homepage: www.tased.edu.au/tasonline/hwhc/hwhc.htm

Victoria
Women's Health Victoria
Level 1, 123 Lonsdale Street
Melbourne VIC 3000
GPO Box 1160K, Melbourne VIC 3001
Phone: 03 9662 3755
Fax: 03 9663 7955
Health information line: 03 9662 3742, 1800 133 321
Email: whv@whv.org.au
Homepage: www.whv.org.au

Western Australia
Women's Health Care House
100 Aberdeen Street
Northbridge WA 6003
Phone: 08 9227 8122, 1800 998 399
Fax: 08 9227 6615
Email: whch@iinet.net.au
Homepage: www.womenshealthwa.iinet.net.au

Index

153

vegetables, recommended intake
  85–6, 103
vegetarians 13, 43, 96
vitamins
  and bone health 122
  for hot flushes 28, 36
  for mood changes 36
water, recommended intake 84,
  107
websites on menopause 139–41
weight loss diets 39
weight-bearing exercise 39,
  43–4, 66
winter foods 97

xanthines 101
X-ray to measure bone density
  42

yoghurt 18, 94, 95, 134
  recommended daily intake
    103
  for vaginal dryness 31

zinc
  absorption 127
  deficiency 126
  recommended intake 96, 127
  role of 126, 127
  sources of 127–8